Prediabetes: A Patient's Guide to Preventing Diabetes

Josie Smythe-Rivers

Table of Contents

Introduction

Prediabetes: A Patient's Guide to Preventing Diabetes is written for those with elevated blood sugar in the prediabetic range who would like to reverse their prediabetes. *Prediabetes* helps you understand the root cause of prediabetes and diabetes, which is insulin resistance. Insulin resistance happens when our cells no longer respond properly to our hormone insulin, which means glucose (sugar) starts accumulating in our blood.

This *Introduction* and subsequent chapters guide you through the reasons we become insulin resistant, and *Prediabetes* gives you the four steps that reverse this condition so you can have normal blood sugar again.

Prediabetes is an early stage of Type 2 diabetes. Current research indicates that even in this early stage prediabetes can cause significant harm to the body. The good news is that you can reverse prediabetes and eliminate your risk of becoming diabetic. The four steps in *Prediabetes: A Patient's Guide to Preventing Diabetes* show you how to become **insulin sensitive** again, which is how we reverse prediabetes.

In addition to the primary focus of this book, which is diet, *Prediabetes* addresses the role exercise, sleep, stress, and appetite play in reversing prediabetes and the insulin resistance causing it. *Prediabetes* also addresses other important insulin-driven conditions including weight gain, high blood pressure, and cholesterol problems.

The reason a book about prediabetes would also address these other common metabolic health problems lies in the fact that each is directly related to the same underlying condition, insulin resistance. As we'll discuss, insulin resistance is *extremely* widespread, but the vast majority of people don't know they're insulin resistant for one reason: we don't get tested for it routinely despite the fact that it's driving all these chronic conditions, including prediabetes and diabetes.

Insulin resistance is behind our population-level, chronic metabolic health epidemics during the last several decades, including diabetes, obesity/weight gain, hypertension, cholesterol problems, nonalcoholic fatty liver disease (NAFLD) as well as many cases of cardiovascular disease and dementia.

Thus, the four steps in *Prediabetes: A Patient's Guide to Preventing Diabetes* that reverse insulin resistance and prediabetes are the same steps that enable us to improve so many related areas of our health—now and for the future. Taking four achievable steps in order to get all these health benefits is an amazing return on one's investment. It may sound impossible that four steps can actually reverse chronic, epidemic metabolic conditions and diseases, but it's true—provided the steps we take address the *actual problem*, which is insulin resistance.

Unfortunately as a culture we've spent decades focused entirely on the wrong things such as counting calories and following dietary advice and guidelines since the 1980's that have significantly *worsened* our blood sugar, weight, and blood pressure, and cholesterol as a population.

Prediabetes: A Patient's Guide to Preventing Diabetes guides you through the reasons prediabetes is a diet-driven hormonal problem and why diet is the *only* effective way to reverse both prediabetes and the insulin resistance causing it. Other lifestyle factors do have an effect on blood sugar and insulin to some degree, especially once we're insulin resistant, so *Prediabetes* also provides you with a functional exercise program that works synergistically with proper diet, adequate sleep, and stress reduction.

Prediabetes: A Patient's Guide to Preventing Diabetes also provides you with guidance about testing your blood sugar at home as an integral part of reversing prediabetes and insulin resistance. *Prediabetes* gives you a concise shopping list of appropriate foods as well as a clear guide to both meal prep and cooking so that you can make many kinds of delicious meals easily and quickly, meals that are key to reversing prediabetes and insulin resistance.
You don't need elaborate meal plans, or hard-to-find ingredients, or "superfoods," etc. because these are not the things that reverse insulin resistance—and because cooking dinner should never look like this humorous video entitled "Perfect One-Pot, 10-Wok, 25-Baking Sheet Dinner" that pokes fun at all those supposedly "easy" weeknight recipes.[1]

The four steps in *Prediabetes* begin with the most important step, the **dietary essentials** in this book that reverse insulin resistance, restore proper levels of appetite, and restore the hormonal signals that tell us when we're full, signals that don't work correctly when we're insulin resistant and have too much circulating insulin in our blood.

This means getting these signals working again through the four steps in *Prediabetes* makes controlling appetite *so much easier*. As we'll discuss, when we're insulin resistant glucose doesn't get into our cells properly, which also means we *become* hungry all the time. Excessive hunger is a *symptom* of insulin resistance as is high blood glucose (sugar)—i.e. prediabetes and diabetes.

---

[1] https://www.youtube.com/watch?v=NGgpSWcaV1U

The other three steps in *Prediabetes* address the effects of sleep, stress, and movement/exercise on insulin levels and blood sugar. When we don't get enough good sleep our hormonal signals don't work properly, and we store more fat.

The activity/exercise program in this book is not about "burning" calories; it's about helping your insulin work properly again as part of reversing prediabetes and the insulin resistance causing it. Finally, the last step is to address stress reduction to the degree you can because stress affects both blood sugar and insulin.

Using This Book

Prediabetes provides you with the metabolic facts about insulin resistance and prediabetes as well as the dietary essentials that reverse these conditions *and* signal satiety *and* build insulin sensitivity. I provide you with a framework for functional exercise that works synergistically with the dietary essentials; I explain the A1C test that measures average blood sugar over time, including the limitations of this test.

I provide you with a program for testing your blood sugar daily as part of charting your progress in reversing prediabetes and insulin resistance. I address the importance of micronutrients from dietary sources, not from supplements, in normalizing blood sugar. I discuss the hormonal effects of exercise, sleep, and stress on insulin and blood sugar.

I also give you pertinent history of dietary changes since the mid-twentieth century that have done such harm to our blood sugar, weight, and blood pressure along with our insulin and cholesterol levels. I address why so much of the dietary and nutritional advice we've received since the 1980's has *worsened* our metabolic health as a population fueling the epidemics of diabetes, obesity, and hypertension.

The wonderful thing about this four-step process of reversing prediabetes and its underlying insulin resistance is that this process is a positive feedback loop; as you start seeing benefits from these taking the steps in this book the process becomes easier, and your results improve more rapidly. Let's get started!

What is Prediabetes?

Technically, prediabetes is not a disease; in 2010 prediabetes became a "diagnostic category." As a diagnostic category prediabetes is actually a vital opportunity to reverse high blood sugar and the insulin resistance causing it by using dietary and lifestyle steps that the data show are more effective than medication. Although prediabetes is defined as a diagnostic category rather than a disease, current research shows that prediabetes does have adverse consequences for multiple areas of our health—even before prediabetes becomes diabetes.

Thus, the actual effects of prediabetes on the body tell us that prediabetes is a disease process rather than simply a diagnostic category; importantly, a diagnosis of prediabetes shows we have a bigger underlying health problem: the insulin resistance that drives high blood sugar as well as a cluster of other metabolic conditions known as "metabolic syndrome," which we will discuss.

It's especially important to understand that prediabetes is one *symptom* of insulin resistance, which is the root cause. Because insulin resistance also drives several related metabolic diseases and conditions that we'll discuss in *Prediabetes: A Patient's Guide to Preventing Diabetes*, other signs of insulin resistance often include hypertension, weight gain, and cholesterol problems. The test that measures average blood sugar, the A1C test, is actually a *belated* reflection of the insulin resistance causing high blood sugar.

This is because insulin resistance usually begins developing long before the symptom of high blood sugar shows up via an A1C test. Yet, prediabetes and the insulin resistance causing it absolutely can be reversed, and in many cases so can Type 2 diabetes—contrary to the myth that Type 2 diabetes is a "progressive" disease.

For many people, reversing prediabetes necessitates losing some weight. The reason for this is that excess weight negatively affects both insulin and blood sugar. Many of us also struggle with managing our weight, blood pressure, and cholesterol.

In most cases these conditions are also due to diet-driven problems with the hormone insulin. The diet that resolves these intertwined chronic metabolic issues isn't complicated or complex—*if we work with the body and not against it*. Unfortunately, the majority of the dietary advice we've been given during the last several decades has been working *against* our metabolic health as the increasing rates of prediabetes, diabetes, hypertension, obesity, and other chronic, diet-driven disease show.

Thus, although prediabetes is the primary subject of this book, we will also discuss these other areas of metabolic health because the cause of high blood sugar, insulin resistance, also drives these other metabolic conditions and because we often we have more than one of these conditions. Therefore, although this book focuses on reversing prediabetes, when you take the four steps in *Prediabetes* you're also going to see significant improvement in managing your blood pressure, weight, and cholesterol.

In addition, by controlling your blood sugar and insulin levels, which *Prediabetes* will teach you how to do, you will also improve your immune health significantly, reduce your risk of certain cancers including liver, colon, pancreas, endometrial, and postmenopausal breast cancer, and significantly reduce your risk of cardiovascular disease and dementia. Controlling blood sugar and insulin levels are *incredibly important* to all areas of our health; and we can do it in four steps.

Logically speaking, advice from nutritional and medical authorities on diet-driven diseases such as prediabetes should *not* make these diet-driven diseases and conditions worse—but that's exactly what's happened since the 1980's. The majority of adults (88%) in the U.S. have one or more chronic metabolic conditions or diseases, which means only 12% of adults are metabolically healthy in terms of blood sugar, weight, blood pressure, and cholesterol levels. *One in every two adults* in the U.S. has or is at risk of having diabetes, and most people with high blood sugar don't know they're prediabetic or even diabetic. Children as young as 3 years old are diagnosed with Type 2 diabetes.

Nearly half of American adults have high blood pressure, which doubles the risk of heart attacks and strokes. 70+% of American adults are either overweight or obese. Up to 85% of American adults may be insulin resistant. A recent article in *Forbes* projects that in a few years we'll be talking about the glucose crisis in the way we now talk about the opioid crisis.[2] As we'll discuss, a significant reason *why* we're so very sick as a population is *because* of the dietary advice we've been following as a nation for the last several decades.

Although our metabolic health, including our blood sugar, is in serious trouble, there is good news too. The way to reverse prediabetes and the underlying insulin resistance causing it as well as so many other related metabolic diseases and conditions is quite straightforward, and the rigorous science tells us this. There are four steps to reversing prediabetes and insulin resistance. In order to help you understand why these four steps work so well, we also need to address what the rigorous science tells us *doesn't* work because we're still surrounded by incorrect dietary and nutritional advice.

Key to reversing prediabetes and insulin resistance is knowing how to avoid all the dietary myths and incorrect advice about blood sugar, diet, weight, and health that are driving the epidemics of diabetes, prediabetes, obesity, hypertension and more—the entire glucose crisis. We'll also address the reasons these myths and bad dietary advice are still so prevalent despite being completely incorrect. In order to reverse prediabetes it's important to be able to recognize incorrect information when you encounter it; and unfortunately we're still inundated by a lot of dietary and nutritional information that is both incorrect and harmful.

---

[2] John Cumbers, "America, Your Diet Is Killing You: Why The Glucose Crisis Will Be Worse Than the Opioid Crisis," *Forbes*, February 17, 2021: https://www.forbes.com/sites/johncumbers/2021/02/17/america-your-diet-is-killing-you-why-the-glucose-crisis-will-be-worse-than-the-opioid-crisis/?sh=6d147d8973d5

Specifics About Prediabetes

Prediabetes is diagnosed when one's A1C test, which measures your average blood sugar over 3 months, falls between 5.7% – 6.4%, and fasting blood glucose lies in the range of 100 – 125 mg/dl. However, blood sugar *below 5.4% is metabolically normal*. Therefore, we should aim to bring our A1C down to 5.4%. An A1C of 5.7 that marks the beginning of the diagnostic category of prediabetes is still too high; prediabetes in this range can still cause vascular damage as well as other types of harm to the body. The data show us this, so it's important to aim for an A1C of 5.4 or below.

Prediabetes is the early stage of Type 2 diabetes, and its effects on the body can be significant—even before prediabetes becomes diabetes. As an early stage of Type 2 diabetes, prediabetes is overwhelmingly a **dietary disease** worsened by 3 things: lack of functional movement (moderate exercise); stress; and sleep deprivation. As a dietary disease driven by consumption of too much carbohydrate over time, including sugar in all forms, prediabetes is often one manifestation of several intertwined metabolic health problems that share the same root cause: insulin resistance.

If one has elevated blood sugar, high blood pressure, cholesterol or weight problems, particularly excess weight around the waistline, this cluster is known as "metabolic syndrome." Within the medical and nutrition science fields these metabolic conditions are said to "cluster;" however, simply describing a "cluster" doesn't address what *causes* the cluster.

The answer is insulin resistance. Most importantly, taking the four steps in *Prediabetes: A Patient's Guide to Preventing Diabetes* enables you to reverse the cluster itself.

The way we reverse these metabolic health problems, including high blood sugar, is by reversing the insulin resistance driving all of them. We do this through diet because diet is the *only* way we can influence the cellular pathways of insulin resistance itself—medications can't do this.

In terms of diet, we reverse insulin resistance by eating *below our carbohydrate tolerance* because carbohydrate is the macronutrient in our diets that drives high blood sugar *and* insulin resistance *and* weight gain *and* hypertension *and* cholesterol problems, especially dangerous triglycerides. In other words, excessive consumption of carbohydrates is causing a severe glucose crisis at the population level. The other two macronutrients in our diet, protein and fat, do not cause any of these metabolic problems, including weight gain.

There is *significantly* more rigorous and robust evidence[3] that carbohydrate restriction is the eating pattern with the best outcomes in treating Type 2 diabetes compared to other eating patterns such as Dash, the Mediterranean diet, or a plant-based eating pattern. The chapter on **dietary essentials** in this book teach you how to identify and eat below your carbohydrate tolerance. We'll also discuss why each person's carbohydrate tolerance is unique and can change over time.

This fact about carbohydrate tolerance—that it's specific to each person—is a key reason many diets and seemingly healthy eating patterns don't work over time in terms of weight loss or blood sugar control or blood pressure control, etc. This is because these eating patterns do not address the causal problem, insulin resistance itself, no matter how "healthy" they seem to be, i.e. no diet except the low-carbohydrate diet addresses the actual reason we develop prediabetes, weight problems, most cases of hypertension, and cholesterol problems—which is because we're becoming increasingly insulin resistant.

Yet, if you have prediabetes, you have a *wonderful opportunity* to prevent worsening of a terrible disease, Type 2 diabetes, and to achieve normal blood sugar again.

---

[3] Hallberg, Sarah J., Dockter, Nancy E., Kushner, Jake A.,,Athinarayanan, Shaminie J. Improving the scientific rigour of nutritional recommendations for adults with type 2 diabetes: A comprehensive review of the American Diabetes Association guideline-recommended eating patters. *Diabetes, Obesity and Metabolism*. 2019 21: 1769-1779: https://doi.org/10.1111/dom.13736

It can be shocking and upsetting to be diagnosed with prediabetes, particularly if you've been eating what we've all been told is a healthy diet. Many medical and dietary authorities will tell you to "cut down on carbs" as the way to address prediabetes. That's the start of the right advice, but it's far too vague.

The reason for this is each person's individual carbohydrate tolerance is different; we need to know which carbs to eliminate, and we need to understand the very important relationship between food timing and insulin levels.

As you'll see in *Prediabetes: A Patient's Guide to Preventing Diabetes,* the most important things we do in order to reverse prediabetes and other insulin-driven health problems are a.) to learn our personal carbohydrate tolerance and b.) eat below that level of carbohydrate tolerance. We'll discuss both of these things in detail.

What Is Insulin Resistance, and Why Does It Cause Prediabetes?

Insulin resistance means our cells no longer take up glucose (sugar) properly from our blood. Most commonly this happens when our cells ignore our hormone insulin as it tries to usher glucose, primarily from the carbohydrate in our diets, into cells to be used for energy. This is just one of the many jobs the hormone insulin has in the human body.

One of the other important jobs insulin has in the body is to prompt fat storage. High insulin levels in the body come from eating above one's carbohydrate tolerance. High insulin levels act like a (hormonal) "lock" trapping fat into our cells so we *can't* release it—i.e. high insulin levels in the blood *prevent* weight loss—and high insulin levels also *prevent* our brains from actually knowing that we're full, which is why we can eat lots of certain kinds of foods, especially refined carbs and sugar, and never feel full. Importantly, calories *are not* related to controlling blood sugar, and calories *do not* govern the process of either gaining or losing weight. These processes are *hormonal*, not caloric.

In addition to insulin resistance driving prediabetes, we can also have a related condition called hyperinsulinemia, which means we have too much insulin in our blood. Insulin resistance causes hyperinsulinemia in most cases; thus, this book treats diet-driven insulin resistance as the primary problem, and the four steps to reversing insulin resistance/prediabetes will address diet-driven hyperinsulinemia as well.

For many people controlling weight is a part of reversing prediabetes as well as an important part of controlling blood pressure and improving so many other areas of health. Thus, it's crucial to understand why weight management, like blood sugar management, is about one thing: *controlling insulin levels in our bodies*, not worrying about calories that have nothing to do with hormones.

As we'll discuss, incorrect dietary and medical advice that "calories" drive health problems, including weight problems and blood sugar problems, is the *single most harmful dietary advice* we've been given in the last several decades for three reasons:

1.) "Calories" don't apply to the human body and never did

2.) Complex metabolic health problems are not caused by simplistic arithmetic; they're due to many complex reasons including hormonal, biochemical, environmental, genetic and epigenetic, reasons

3.) Widespread levels of insulin resistance as a population—and therefore our widespread levels of pre/diabetes and obesity in particular—are due to the ways in which our very recent diet high in carbohydrate (especially sugar) is incompatible with our entire evolution as a species.

For reason that we'll discuss, our evolution as humans plays a key role in why humans have a carbohydrate tolerance level in the first place. We also have a limit to our tolerance for protein, but humans naturally understand and eat at or below our level of protein tolerance. Humans have a much harder time eating at or below our carbohydrate tolerance, which we'll address.

Unlike protein or carbohydrate, the third macronutrient in the human diet is the one for which we have *a far higher tolerance*. That macronutrient is *fat*. That might sound strange, but it's true! Since the 1960's we've misunderstood both carbs and fat and how they affect the body.

Now we do know how carbohydrate and fat affect the human body; the problem is that inaccurate beliefs and narratives about carbohydrate and fat are still incredibly pervasive because we've been hearing them for decades.

The rigorous science tells us clearly how fat and carbohydrate affect the body, which we will discuss; but widespread beliefs about carbohydrate and fat within nutrition science as well as in medical institutions and education remain decades out of date. This means we're still surrounded by the wrong information and dietary advice, which is why prediabetes, diabetes, obesity, hypertension, NAFLD and other chronic metabolic conditions and diseases keep getting worse, not better.

Why We're Still Getting the Wrong Dietary and Nutritional Advice

In terms of reversing prediabetes, this may sound strange that we're still being given the wrong information. It may sound surprising that the very institutions and dietary authorities that should be the most aware of the rigorous evidence are often so out of date; however, it takes generations for paradigms (belief systems) to shift.

For example, we may look back with astonishment at the fact that Sir Isaac Newton, inventor of calculus and the "father" of modern physics, actually spent much of his life practicing alchemy. Although it may sound bizarre to us that he would believe in such a thing, belief in alchemy was a prominent paradigm in his time. It was a way of trying to understand the secrets of nature prior to the invention of what we now know as the scientific method as well as the scientific instruments we have today.

We no longer believe in alchemy as paradigm or as a way of understanding the complexities of nature; we know we can't take base metals such as lead and turn them into gold; however, many of the things Newton learned while trying to transform these base metals into gold actually helped him develop his conceptual framework regarding action-at-a distance—i.e. gravity.

Thus, in the long sweep of history it's not surprising that we too have spent several decades believing the wrong paradigms about diet and nutrition—for example, believing that fat makes us fat and that carbohydrate is good for us at high levels. These beliefs are as incorrect as alchemy was, but like Newton we can use incorrect dietary beliefs and paradigms to help us get to the *right dietary paradigms* that reverse prediabetes, diabetes, and obesity.

Newton had to invent calculus in order to describe the right paradigms about nature; fortunately for us the science is already giving us the rigorous evidence (the right paradigms) about how carbohydrate and fat actually affect our bodies, most especially our blood sugar.

As a field nutrition science has spent decades thinking in ways that resemble alchemy, not science, i.e. believing that fat makes us fat, that carbohydrate makes us healthy and that we must eat lots of it or we won't have enough energy. For decades the governing paradigm about weight loss has been that we must "burn" more calories than we consume.

These beliefs are incorrect—just as it's not true that we can turn lead into gold—no matter how much we might believe we can. Alchemy made sense to Newton in his time for a number of reasons, just as the above ideas have made sense to us since the 1980's. However, "making sense" and actually *being accurate* are different things.

In discussing the reason carbohydrate restriction is the only dietary method of reversing prediabetes and its underlying cause, insulin resistance, we'll also address some of the evolutionary history of the human body. This discussion is to help you better understand how carbohydrate, protein, fat, and insulin affect the body so you can see why so much standard dietary and medical advice about blood sugar and weight problems is actually nonsensical and has been for decades—as nonsensical as alchemy.

The reason much of the dietary advice we're still being given is nonsensical is twofold. First, the reason we develop prediabetes, diabetes, weight gain, cholesterol problems and so many other metabolic diseases lies in our evolutionary history, specifically in the way the hormone insulin works, which we'll discuss.

Second, for decades we've been advised to eat a diet high in carbohydrate, including plenty of "whole grains," despite the fact that carbohydrate, unlike fat or protein, is the only macronutrient that raises blood sugar and insulin levels significantly, causing us to develop the insulin resistance over time that drives blood sugar problems.

For decades the prevailing dietary paradigm has been that it's actually healthy to eat this diet *that drives pre/diabetes, obesity, cholesterol problems, etc*. Eating this diet is akin to trying to turn base metals (i.e. a bad diet that causes insulin resistance) into the gold of good health. Like alchemy, this diet doesn't work, and it never did. It's made our health much worse—much like practicing alchemy often poisoned alchemists as they tried to turn toxic substances into gold. We can't turn a toxic diet into good health—which is what we've been told we can do since the 1980's.

Although prediabetes is overwhelmingly a dietary disease, genetics can play a role within families regarding tendencies toward metabolic health issues that can include high blood sugar, weight gain, high blood pressure, and cholesterol problems. However, genetics are *not* the main reason these metabolic health problems actually develop: diet is the main reason.

If we have a genetic tendency toward any of these metabolic problems, we must use proper diet as the *powerful* medical tool that it is in order to manage, and in many cases, reverse these conditions. Culturally we're accustomed to thinking of diet as secondary to genetics; it's not.

What's Evolution Got To Do With It?

Diet has very powerful effects on gene expression in terms of turning many genes on or off. As we'll also discuss, throughout our evolutionary history as a species diet was crucial to how the majority of our genes were established; our diet during this evolutionary history (millions of years) is also key to how the human body still works—especially with regard to blood sugar and insulin.

For example, as we'll discuss diet can *change* what the human body uses as its source of energy. That's very powerful! Think of it this way, we live modern lives, but the way our bodies work is *ancient*, and we'll discuss why our modern diets are so profoundly incompatible with our evolutionary history—an incompatibility that is *causing* epidemic levels of pre/diabetes, obesity, hypertension, and other metabolic problems.

The link between our evolutionary history and current diet-driven diseases such as pre/diabetes, weight problems, blood pressure problems etc. lies in *how diet affects the hormone insulin*. We tend to think of fossils as evidence of the past—especially of the ancient past; however, as you'll see it's actually the hormone insulin that connects our evolutionary past to our current chronic metabolic health crisis globally, including the high rates of prediabetes and diabetes.

Thus, the way our diet affects the hormone insulin is ancient and extremely powerful. This also means each of us has enormous power to use diet to reverse the diet-driven insulin resistance causing prediabetes as well as other insulin-related metabolic health problems.

The power of diet in our evolution as a species *and in how our bodies still work to this day* is profound; however, equally important is the way in which our current access to foods and healthcare determines many of our options regarding diet.

Specific population groups also have a propensity to develop prediabetes and diabetes at higher rates due to social and cultural forces that include food deserts in which *un*processed and *un*refined foods are difficult to find as well as unequal access to healthcare.

Thus, controlling blood sugar can be more difficult for some people for reasons we don't necessarily control, including both genetic tendencies and current forms of structural and social inequality. However, taking the four steps in *Prediabetes* works for everyone. Let's discuss these four steps.

The Four Steps

Using both scientific and historical frameworks, *Prediabetes* will help you understand the best choices to make regarding diet, exercise, sleep, and stress so that you can reverse prediabetes within the circumstances you have. The four steps in this book work for *everyone* because they are based in current, rigorous science, not social narratives, cultural beliefs, or the unscientific nonsense that dominates much of nutritional "science" as a field.

Some of us will need to focus on one or two of these four steps more than the other steps, and we'll discuss why this is the case. Similarly, the low-carb eating options regarding the diet that reverses prediabetes exist on a *continuum*, so you can make the choices that are feasible and appropriate for you. We will discuss these choices throughout *Prediabetes: A Patient's Guide to Preventing Diabetes*.

Reversing prediabetes means taking these four steps consistently, but we also need flexibility in order to be consistent in reaching the only outcome that reverses prediabetes: that outcome is achieving **insulin sensitivity**. Restoring our insulin sensitivity is a process; once we've restored our insulin sensitivity, these same four steps prevent insulin resistance from returning.

As we restore insulin sensitivity we're *also* controlling weight, blood pressure, and cholesterol levels at the same time, which we will discuss. By far the two most important factors that restore insulin sensitivity, reverse insulin resistance, and reverse prediabetes are what we eat and when we eat.

What We Eat and When We Eat

The single *most important step* in reversing prediabetes is to eat a diet that minimizes blood sugar and insulin spikes—i.e. a diet low in carbohydrate. Both what we eat and when we eat determine our blood sugar, insulin levels, and weight—more than any other factors. It's important to understand that reversing prediabetes means paying attention to *both* what we eat *and when we eat*, which is called food timing.

Often nutritional and dietary advice regarding prediabetes and diabetes tells us to snack in order to "keep up" our energy and keep our blood sugar "stable." *This is absolutely wrong*; as we'll discuss, snacking is a serious problem if you have prediabetes (or diabetes) because *snacking worsens insulin resistance* over time—the insulin resistance that causes prediabetes/diabetes in the first place. We'll discuss this dangerous myth that snacking helps keep blood sugar "stable."

The low-carbohydrate diet that minimizes blood sugar and insulin spikes is also the same diet that controls weight, blood pressure, and cholesterol. We don't need, nor should we try, multiple diets to control blood sugar, or weight, or blood pressure, or cholesterol. We definitely should not cycle between diets; we need the correct eating pattern that reverses high blood sugar as well as other metabolic health problems that are rooted in diet-driven insulin resistance.

The chapter on **dietary essentials in this book** gives you the eating plan that reverses diet-driven insulin resistance with flexible choices contingent upon your blood sugar and level of insulin resistance. As we've noted, we also need flexibility to determine what works for each of us because each of us has a different level of carbohydrate tolerance.

Why Calories Are Nonsense, and Why "Willpower" Is Not the Issue

"Calories" are irrelevant to controlling blood sugar, appetite, and weight. The reason for this is that calories do not cause high blood sugar, or insulin resistance, or weight gain; quantity of food (i.e. how much we eat) is relevant, but quantity is not the same thing as "calories," and we'll discuss this important difference. Far more important is *what we eat* in terms of the ratio of the 3 macronutrients (protein, carbohydrate, and fat) as well as *when we eat*.

In fact, we're often driven to eat too much *because* we're insulin resistant and prediabetic. Once we fix the actual problem—insulin resistance and having too much insulin in our blood—appetite becomes far more predictable and manageable, and food cravings decrease significantly. The quantity of food we eat decreases naturally as insulin levels normalize. This process has nothing to do with calories; it's a hormonal process, and it's not related to willpower.

This may sound strange because we're constantly told to worry about calories and to "burn" more "energy" than we consume, which is the current euphemism for talking about calorie reduction—i.e. for talking about calories without saying the word "calories" and talking vaguely about "energy" instead. *All calorie-based advice is the wrong advice* because "calories" are the wrong framework (paradigm) for talking about hormones and biochemistry. The idea that eating too many "calories" causes weight gain and problems with blood sugar is not accurate either mathematically or at any other level.

As we've noted, the chief reason "calories" are not relevant to blood sugar or weight management is because prediabetes and weight problems are *hormonal problems, not caloric ones*.
In following the **dietary essentials in this book**, you may even eat *more* calories and *more fat* as part of *losing weight*, and we'll address how this works.

Remember, we can't lose weight until insulin is no longer "locking" down our fat cells and preventing them from releasing fat—and being overweight does negatively affect blood sugar, so it's important to address the cause of weight problems—high levels of insulin.

Cutting calories *never tells* insulin to stop locking down the fat in our cells. Lowering your intake of carbohydrate tells insulin levels to go down and to stop locking fat in—i.e. lowering carbohydrate tells insulin *to let the fat out* of the cells. It may seem strange to think of a hormone such as insulin as a "lock," but that's essentially how it works. We'll discuss this in further detail.

Once our blood sugar and insulin levels are out of balance, our hunger/appetite *increases*. These imbalances in blood sugar and insulin levels then *cause* us to eat and drink the wrong things, especially sugar and other starchy foods, and to eat too much and too often. We'll address the reasons for this in subsequent sections of this book.

Yet, the belief that appetite is a matter of willpower is still deeply entrenched in standard medical, dietary, and nutritional advice. This belief is *incorrect*; it's dogma, not science. Managing appetite is all about reversing insulin resistance and controlling our blood sugar.

Once we do both, appetite normalizes significantly. This happens automatically. The reason is that "willpower" to cut calories or exercise for long periods is no match for the incredibly powerful hormone insulin. "Willpower" may be highly valued personality trait, but it's an abstract concept that's cultural and social, not hormonal. It's a *narrative* we use in many different ways and for many different reasons.

Think of the difference between "willpower" and insulin this way: you show up to a tennis game on a beautiful sunny day, and because you have lots of "willpower" to play well, you feel confident. However, your tennis partner shows up with one of those automatic machines (insulin in this analogy) and begins firing tennis balls at you with astonishing accuracy and at a terrifying rate. This is not a fair match.

No matter how much "willpower" you have, you're going to lose this tennis match because you're up against impossible odds. Like the machine in this analogy, our hormone insulin is extremely powerful; it does many jobs in the body, and it does them very accurately and rapidly. In this analogy, the machine firing tennis balls at you will prevail; willpower is no match for it, just as willpower is no match for insulin.

If we encountered this situation on the tennis court, we'd know immediately that we couldn't prevail, and we'd find another tennis partner. We wouldn't keep playing thinking that we could outrun and outplay a machine forever. Eventually we'd have to stop.

The problem is that most dietary advice since the 1980's has been telling us to stay on the court and that we can beat a far more powerful force, the insulin resistance causing weight gain and blood sugar problems as well as other metabolic health issues. We've been told we can overcome insulin-driven prediabetes and other health problems by doing stuff that *doesn't work* such as having more "willpower," reducing enough "calories," not eating fat or meat, and increasing our intake of carbohydrate, which causes our insulin resistance in the first place.

Like the machine firing tennis balls at us in this analogy, *insulin* is controlling the game. That's why the four steps in this book are about restoring insulin sensitivity—because that's all that matters.

High blood sugar and weight gain are *symptoms* of insulin resistance, which is a hormonal problem; diabetes, prediabetes, weight gain, hypertension, etc. do *not* reflect willpower, or character, or morals, or how much we reduce calories, etc. These have been the predominant narratives about weight problems in particular since the middle of the nineteenth century.

They are *narratives*, and they are incorrect. Excessive hunger is a very clear sign of worsening insulin resistance—it's a symptom, not a cause. Once we address the fundamental problem, insulin resistance, the symptoms of high blood sugar and excessive hunger and weight gain abate.

It is accurate that prediabetes and diabetes are very strongly linked to being overweight; however, people with a normal BMI can also have prediabetes and/or insulin resistance. In other words, prediabetes, diabetes, and weight problems are all manifestations of insulin resistance; however, not everyone who is insulin resistant and/or prediabetic is overweight.

Some people who are insulin resistant are prediabetic but not overweight; some people who are insulin resistant have high blood pressure but normal blood sugar. Thus, people differ in terms of the specific manifestations of insulin resistance that they experience—but our symptoms will worsen over time if we don't address the underlying insulin resistance itself.

Thus, in terms of managing blood sugar and/or weight and/or blood pressure, there is one thing on which we have to focus: stabilizing insulin secretion in the body, which this book teaches you how to do. There is also one thing on which we should not focus: calories.

The reason calories are nonsensical when it comes to either blood sugar and weight management is that our cells and genes and organs can't count, so they have no idea what calories are. This sounds very silly, but the entire assumption behind calories is that the human body and all its complex biochemical and hormonal processes are somehow drive by simple arithmetic.

This idea is as nonsensical as alchemy, and it always has been. Calories have come to *seem* normal to us because the *narrative* of calories in/calories out has repeated for decades, and because it's a narrative that *seems* to be objective because it uses arithmetic.

We inherited the idea of "calories" from other scientific and technological fields in the nineteenth century. The construct of calories *is* applicable in these other fields; however, *calories do not apply to the human body*, and they never did. In the early twentieth century, nutrition science transposed this idea of "calories" (energy) from these other fields to the human body.

Nutrition science essentially took the *idea* of "calories" from other applicable fields and turned it into a *metaphor* for energy vis-à-vis the human body. However, the human body doesn't have any receptors for calories, so when we eat or drink something the body does not metabolize these things according to "calories." *The body has no way of recognizing calories*. It's a metaphor that doesn't work. The human body recognizes protein, fat, and carbohydrate.

So, while we've spent decades worrying about calories as a population we've become far more sick with chronic metabolic diseases such as obesity, pre/diabetes, hypertension, and cholesterol problems—and their downstream conditions such as cardiovascular disease—because we've been focused on the wrong thing: "calories" that the human body does not recognize at the biochemical, metabolic, or any other level. Yet we haven't been focused on what causes prediabetes and diabetes and obesity and other chronic health problems: insulin resistance.

Millions of people go on all types of diets every year in order to control blood sugar and weight; yet more than 70% of American adults are obese or overweight—and it's *not* because we aren't trying to lose weight as a population. This fact alone makes it very clear that reducing calories doesn't work and cutting out fat doesn't work.

We've done these things for decades, and prediabetes, diabetes and obesity are getting worse. If cutting calories and avoiding fat actually worked we wouldn't need to try multiple diets, and we wouldn't regain the weight as we almost always do.

Reducing the "calories" of what we consume, and reducing fat, are not the *mechanisms* through which we address weight, or blood sugar, or blood pressure, or cholesterol problems—if they were, all these chronic metabolic conditions and diseases wouldn't be getting worse year after year.

Just to review for a moment, the way we reverse these metabolic health problems, including high blood sugar, is by reversing the insulin resistance driving them. Insulin resistance means our cells no longer take up glucose (sugar) from the blood effectively because our cells are ignoring the hormone insulin when it attempts to usher glucose into cells to be used for energy, which is one of the many jobs insulin does in the body.

We may also have a related condition called hyperinsulinemia, which means we have too much insulin in our blood. Insulin resistance causes hyperinsulinemia in most cases, so this book focuses on reversing diet-driven insulin resistance. Now let's discuss the relationship between the macronutrient carbohydrate and insulin resistance, which causes prediabetes.

A Diet High In Carbohydrate Causes Insulin Resistance, Which Drives Prediabetes

The diet responsible for insulin resistance and therefore prediabetes and weight gain is the standard American diet, which is comprised of 60% highly processed foods and drinks as well as far too much carbohydrate in general, especially sugar in all forms, including juice.

This standard American diet causes the insulin resistance that's responsible for pre/diabetes as well as uncontrolled hypertension across multiple populations, obesity, and widespread problems with cholesterol. This is because the carbohydrate-centered standard American diet quickly *becomes* a huge amount of sugar inside the human body, which automatically drives up insulin secretion, blood sugar, and blood pressure—before getting stored as fat.

We might be eating foods with no "added" sugar, which is a good start; but we need to pay *as much attention to foods that become sugar in our bodies*. What nutrition fact labels on products tell us is limited, frequently inaccurate, and often misleading. Ingredient lists are worse because companies manipulate them to make their products appear to be healthy when they are definitely not healthy—for example, using **50+ terms/names for sugar**[4] in order to hide how bad these products are for our blood sugar and insulin levels.

All these diseases, including prediabetes, are driven by one macronutrient in our diet, carbohydrate. The other way of saying this is that as a culture we're *exposed* to chronic carbohydrate toxicity, most especially in processed foods, refined grains and flours, and sugar in a bewildering range of forms, both natural and artificial. All these supposedly "whole grains" we're constantly told to eat *also drive* the insulin resistance over time that's causing epidemic levels

---

[4] Barnwell, Anna. "Secret Sugars: The 56 Different Names for Sugar." Virta Blog. December, 2018: https://www.virtahealth.com/blog/names-for-sugar

of prediabetes and diabetes.

Anything can be called a "whole grain," which is not a scientific term or phrase, and most of this stuff is anything but whole grain. This toxic level of carbohydrate exposure is driving insulin resistance across the population, and evidence suggests that 85% of American adults may be insulin resistant to some degree. (We don't know the percentage exactly because people aren't tested routinely for insulin resistance, but other reliable data point to this very high level of insulin resistance at the population level.)

This means that insulin resistance is increasing even faster than diabetes across the globe. Without consistent, routine testing for insulin resistance just like cholesterol and blood pressure testing, downstream metabolic conditions and diseases, including prediabetes, diabetes, obesity, and cardiovascular disease, will continue to worsen—and they're *already at epidemic levels*.

When one or more of these downstream conditions shows up such as hypertension, prediabetes, obesity, cardiovascular disease, etc., people *still* aren't tested for insulin resistance; therefore, we're not being told how *severe* our insulin resistance is or how to reverse this fundamental problem driving all these diseases. We don't need to be overweight to be insulin resistant; weight gain is one symptom, which not everyone gets. There are some rare exceptions, but if we are overweight it's almost always certain that we have insulin resistance to some degree. If we are prediabetic we are insulin resistant.

Yet, despite the epidemic levels of chronic metabolic diseases and conditions, including high blood sugar, insulin resistance remains primarily a subject of research interest, not clinical practice, which must change. My book *Metabolic Health: Prediabetes, Diabetes, Insulin Resistance, and Weight Loss* (ASIN : B07W98PCMG) contains a chapter dedicated to testing, including blood sugar and insulin resistance testing, if you would like further guidance on getting tested for insulin resistance.

Protein and Fat

Keep in mind that the other two macronutrients in our diet, protein and fat, do not cause metabolic diseases and conditions, including the insulin resistance that drives pre/diabetes, obesity and high blood pressure. For decades we've been told that eating fat makes us fat and that saturated fat in particular hurts our heart health; this is the *paradigm* we've inherited, and it's incorrect.

For decades the unproven idea was that dietary fat and cholesterol "clog" the arteries leading to cardiovascular disease. Atherosclerosis, hardening of the arteries, is an inflammatory problem, not one of "clogged" arteries. The human vascular system does not resemble drainpipes!

The current, robust science in the last decade does not support the notion that if we eat fat it just accumulates in our arteries. In fact, it's becoming clearer that fat from natural sources such as butter, cheese, meat, fatty fish, etc. has *protective* benefits for the heart. These natural fats do not include "vegetable" oils such as corn, soybean, canola, etc., which are *incredibly* toxic and harm cardiovascular health—they are not natural—they are light machine oils that are made through intensive chemical and industrial processes.

Incorrect cultural narratives and myths about natural sources of saturated fat in particular are very powerful, so it will take time for the culture (as well as dieticians and doctors) to see natural sources of fat correctly—i.e. *the natural fats on which we evolved as a species*. This is important because the less fat we eat, the more carbohydrate we tend to eat—i.e. the macronutrient that's actually causing the weight gain and prediabetes in the first place.

Carbohydrate toxicity causes us to develop high triglycerides, a type of fat that does damage the heart. It's not the fat in the diet that harms the heart—it's the carbs turning into this type of fat that hurts our heart health.

By limiting intake of fat over the last several decades we've increased our consumption of carbohydrate *significantly*, especially refined and processed carbs; the decades in which our metabolic health problems became epidemics are the same decades in which we have lowered intake of fat and increased the amount of carbohydrate we eat.

Humans *can't survive* without either protein *or* fat, and telling us to eat a diet high in carbohydrate, which causes insulin resistance and diabetes, as well light machine oils such as corn, soybean, cottonseed, etc., is incredibly dangerous—but it's dietary advice that very good for agribusiness profits, processed food industries, and drug companies. These entities are *major* contributors to diet-related research, medical and nutritional education and institutions, nonprofit health organizations, etc., so we're most often get dietary and nutritional advice filtered through these economic priorities and pressures.

As we'll discuss, not all carbohydrates are the same in terms of their effect on blood sugar, insulin levels, weight, and cholesterol; however, as a population it is factually the case that we eat far more carbohydrate, most especially in processed and refined forms, than the human body was designed through millions of years of evolution to tolerate—resulting in chronic metabolic diseases and conditions across nearly the entire population, in all age groups, for the first time in human history.

This high carbohydrate diet also *starves our bodies* of essential vitamins and minerals (micronutrients). Obesity is endemic in the U.S. and increasing globally. Especially troubling is the fact that nutritional deficiencies and obesity often occur together. To reverse prediabetes, you must eliminate sugar, including juice, as well as simple, refined, and processed carbohydrate (e.g. grains and flours), which we will discuss.

This is what most MD's mean when they say, "cut down on the carbs." Keep in mind that MD's get basically no training in nutrition; only about 20% of medical schools require any training in nutrition despite the fact that food has extraordinarily powerful effects on every aspect of our bodies, including our genes.

As a field, nutrition science promotes a carbohydrate-centered diet for reasons that lie in social, economic, and cultural pressures—not because carbohydrate is inherently healthy; that's the myth. Our national dietary guidelines, *Dietary Guidelines for Americans,*[5] promotes consumption of enormous amounts of carbohydrate, which raises blood sugar and insulin levels, especially all those "whole grains" we're told to eat for reasons that lie in stubborn cultural paradigms about carbohydrate and fat, politics, economics, ideology, and *a lot* of industry-funded junk masquerading as nutrition "science."

At the same time, these Guidelines have claimed for decades that saturated fat is bad for our health—which is just a hypothesis, one that has never been proven despite *enormous* sums of money having been spent for decades trying to do so. The belief, the paradigm, that saturated fat is bad for us is perhaps the most studied hypothesis in nutrition science; yet robust evidence doesn't support the dogmatic belief that dietary fat, including saturated fat, is bad for us.

Despite all the evidence that alchemy didn't work, people, including Newton, believed in it for centuries. This is the situation in which we find ourselves regarding both fat and carbohydrate vis-à-vis the evidence.

---

[5] U.S. Department of Agriculture and U.S. Department of Health and Human Services. Dietary Guidelines for Americans, 2020-2025. 9th Edition. December 2020. Available at DietaryGuidelines.gov

Reversing Your Prediabetes

So "cut down on the carbs" is the beginning of the answer to reversing prediabetes; reversing prediabetes actually means addressing the four factors that are the subject of this book:

1.) Diet: specifically eating *below your personal carbohydrate tolerance* and *controlling food timing*, both of **which this book addresses in detail**

2.) Increasing **functional exercise** through the program in this book helps you restore your insulin sensitivity by helping insulin work better in your body; it's not about "burning" calories

3.) **Increasing sleep** if you're sleep deprived as addressed in the chapter on sleep deprivation in this book

4.) **Decreasing stress** to the degree you can because stress has hormonal effects on the body, which we'll discuss

Along with the dietary changes that we'll discuss in detail, getting enough activity/exercise as well as enough sleep will significantly accelerate this process of reversing prediabetes by stabilizing both blood sugar and insulin levels.

The byproduct of taking the four steps above will be safe weight loss so that you don't gain it back, and we'll address the differences between safe/permanent weight loss—and temporarily tricking your body into weight loss through calorie-reduction diets. Exercise, sleep, and stress reduction are not just generic "lifestyle" factors; each affects our blood sugar and our insulin levels directly—and over time, they help us restore insulin sensitivity.

However, you don't need to exercise for hours a day to control either blood sugar or weight. This is because burning calories is *not* the point; restoring *insulin sensitivity* is the point. Restoring insulin sensitivity through the four steps above is what reverses prediabetes and enables us both to lose weight and *keep it off*. We experience repeated failure on diets not because we don't "stick" to them but because the diets are wrong. They don't address the problem, which is insulin resistance and hyperinsulinemia.

As we've been discussing, calories and hormones are *very* different things; however, as a culture we've been focused entirely on "calories" for decades despite the fact that calories are not what cause prediabetes, or weight gain, or high blood sugar, or cardiovascular disease, or low HDL/high triglycerides.

These conditions and diseases are all manifestations of carbohydrate-driven insulin resistance—**carbohydrate toxicity**. In other words, if you have any of these conditions or diseases, you're experiencing carbohydrate toxicity, which is causing problems with the hormone insulin in your body.

The word "toxicity" may sound a bit extreme, but keep in mind that we can become very sick if we eat protein to toxic levels, or if we drink water to toxic levels. As a species we're not designed through millions of years of evolution to consume anything to toxic levels—including things that are good for us at normal and safe levels such as protein and water.

Yet, we've been *told* for decades that everyone *should* eat carbohydrate to toxic levels *and* avoid natural sources of fat that are *essential* to our survival and health. The reasons we've been told this are complex historically, and we'll discuss some of them.

The main thing to understand is that carbohydrate is an *optional* macronutrient in the human diet; it is not essential, which means it's not necessary for us to eat carbohydrate the way both protein and fat are necessary for both health and survival. This doesn't mean you shouldn't eat any carbs; it means we have *a lot more choice about eating carbohydrates* than we've been told for reasons that lie in corporate profits, bias, ideological-driven dietary advice, and a lot of very sloppy research in nutrition science as a field.

Let's return for a moment to the issue of calories and why counting them is beside the point when it comes to weight loss, prediabetes, or any other metabolic condition. As noted above, the reason for this is because the human body has no receptors for "calories." "Calories" are not the "language" the body understands. The "language" of the human body is hormonal, not caloric. By focusing on calories as a culture essentially we've been speaking the *wrong language* to the body. To reverse prediabetes we have to think in the language the body understands. That language is protein, fat, and carbohydrate, the 3 macronutrients in relation to each other—how much of each macronutrient we eat—and when we eat these macronutrients.

Nutrition fact labels on products put calories in a bigger, bold font at the top—that's the visual equivalent of yelling at someone in a different language; yelling doesn't change the problem, which is a language difference—i.e. raising volume of speech doesn't increase comprehension. No matter how large the font, it's not going to change the fact that "calories" don't apply to the human body, to our weight, our blood sugar, or anything else. Our bodies don't understand them because they have no means (mechanism) for doing so.

A Closer Look At Carbohydrate

Why is the macronutrient carbohydrate, rather than protein or fat, the overwhelming problem in terms of prediabetes and insulin resistance? Carbohydrate is what becomes glucose (sugar) in our blood, sugar the body either has to *use* for energy, or *store* as fat because humans can't store carbohydrate directly. (Protein also turns into glucose, but at a far lower level—i.e. it's a distant second in terms of raising blood sugar and insulin levels.)

Fat does not raise blood sugar. Fat does not raise insulin levels. Eating a diet high in carbohydrate causes prolonged, severe, and damaging spikes in blood sugar and insulin secretion, which happen together.

Over time, sometimes as long as two decades, these constant spikes multiple times a day—and over long periods of time each day if we snack—cause insulin resistance and hyperinsulinemia, which show up downstream as prediabetes, weight gain, hypertension, cholesterol issues, and later as cardiovascular disease as well as other diet-driven conditions such as dementia because the brain is exquisitely sensitive to chronic high blood sugar.

In response to these constant spikes in blood sugar and insulin, cells start to ignore insulin when it tries to push more glucose into them. When our cells no longer respond to insulin trying to usher more glucose into them, which is one of the jobs insulin does in our bodies, that sugar begins to pool up in the blood. When we are insulin resistant glucose (sugar) pools up in the blood because it's not getting into our cells to be used for energy. This forces the pancreas to keep pumping out more insulin, which is our fat storage hormone.

High levels of insulin mean increased fat storage. As we've mentioned, high levels of insulin "lock down" the fat in the cells so we can't lose weight. Because our cells also aren't getting the energy they need, we become hungry more easily, and we eat more.

Sometimes our cells are not yet insulin resistant, but because they already have too much glucose in them from a diet high in carbohydrate, they can't take any more in. We can have both problems.

To summarize: in the majority of cases insulin resistance causes prediabetes. Some individuals also have hyperinsulinemia as well, which is when we have too much insulin in the blood. Both are caused by a diet that's far too high in the one macronutrient in our diet that is entirely optional, carbohydrate, most especially in foods/drinks that are processed and refined—i.e. juices/sodas, grains, flours, starches—sugar in all forms, *including* artificial and alternative sweeteners that can still spike insulin levels even if they don't spike blood sugar directly.

Thus, the way we reverse prediabetes is to correct insulin resistance and hyperinsulinemia *via diet* so we become insulin sensitive again. The two dietary steps are a.) controlling intake of carbohydrate, most especially in processed forms, and b.) using food timing to control blood sugar *and* insulin levels. These two dietary steps are all about hormones, not calories.

Exercise helps insulin usher glucose into the cells instead of prompting our bodies to store all this excess sugar from a high carbohydrate diet as fat; when glucose gets used by our muscles for energy instead of being stored as fat, we begin to release fat—weight loss. Adequate sleep and stress reduction help restore normal blood sugar through other hormonal processes. Cutting "calories" cannot address a hormonal problem.

Further, as we'll discuss calorie-reduction diets, no matter what they're actually called, often worsen both blood sugar and insulin resistance by slowing your metabolism, which is a *serious problem* for many reasons.

Your healthcare team may tell you to lose weight if you need to do so in order to improve your blood sugar. Excess weight negatively affects blood sugar; however, excess weight, like high blood sugar, *is a manifestation*—a symptom of insulin resistance. We correct weight problems and high blood sugar by fixing the insulin resistance underlying both.

Your healthcare team may tell you that the way to lose weight is to reduce calories (i.e. balance "energy" intake with "energy" expenditure—which is now the more euphemistic/fashionable way of talking about calories.) All this sounds vaguely mathematical and objective, and it's repeated so often we think it's correct. It's wrong, and there are *serious* long-term consequences of cutting calories.

Cutting calories and eating below your carbohydrate tolerance are two *very different things*. The difference between them is how they affect insulin, which is what matters. Calories don't cause weight gain or high blood sugar; insulin resistance and having too much insulin (the fat storage hormone) circulating in the body cause weight gain, which in turn worsens blood sugar. Think of it this way: we do not gain weight because we're eating too much; we eat too much because we're gaining weight—i.e. because we are insulin resistant.

Thus, calories are not the issue when it comes either to weight loss or controlling blood sugar because calories don't solve a hormonal problem. Calories and hormones are entirely different things, but as a culture we've been confusing them for decades—as prediabetes, obesity, diabetes, and other metabolic health problems have gotten far worse.

They've gotten far worse *because* we haven't been testing for insulin resistance at the population level and because people have been told to focus on "calories" *and* eat a high carbohydrate diet, including a lot of "whole grains" and sugary fruits, etc. that spike blood sugar and insulin levels repeatedly.

In addition to eating a low carbohydrate diet, as part of reversing insulin resistance we also need to increase our exercise/movement in order to help insulin work better in our bodies, reduce chronic stress as much as possible because it floods the body with cortisol, which we'll discuss, and get enough sleep because chronic sleep deprivation affects insulin as well as blood sugar directly, and it is strongly associated with weight gain.

Thus, as we've been discussing, prediabetes is one manifestation of insulin resistance, which is a diet-driven hormonal problem caused by excessive (toxic) carbohydrate consumption; lack of movement, poor sleep, and far too much stress also contribute to high blood sugar for reasons that are hormonal, not caloric. Finally, given the increasing rate of obesity, prediabetes, and diabetes among young people, as a population and as a species we're experiencing carbohydrate toxicity at younger and younger ages.

As insulin resistance worsens over time, prediabetes suddenly becomes Type 2 diabetes; prediabetes goes along for a while as prediabetes, but typically there's a sudden jump to diabetes due to worsening insulin resistance. Insulin resistance also plays a decisive role in many other diseases and conditions such as cardiovascular disease, nonalcoholic fatty liver disease (NAFLD), dementia, infertility, erectile dysfunction, and other conditions.

Therefore, insulin resistance is a serious condition that has multiple effects throughout the entire human body. It's a condition that negatively affects the entire body including blood sugar. Unfortunately, most people are never tested for insulin resistance along with other routine tests such as blood pressure, weight, and cholesterol levels. We're tested for the downstream diseases and conditions caused by insulin resistance—but not for the insulin resistance itself.

The good news is that with the dietary and lifestyle changes we'll discuss, the four steps of this book, you can reverse insulin resistance and become **insulin sensitive** again. This means you'll be improving multiple areas of your metabolic health at the same time, including blood sugar, blood pressure, cholesterol, and weight.

Even better—you don't need hard-to-find foods, questionable supplements, expensive meal plans, or nonsense of any sort! These things don't work because they don't reverse the actual problem, the underlying insulin resistance. (They're very profitable, but they don't work—which is what makes them profitable—i.e. because these things don't work, people end up blaming themselves for "failure," and they have to keep trying different things.)

The reason these things don't work is because *diet is the only way we influence the cellular pathways of insulin resistance*. There are no "superfoods," or magic vitamins, or calorie-restriction diets, *or medications* that can do this. This is because reversing prediabetes is not about any of this stuff. Specifically, only a diet low in carbohydrate positively influences these cellular pathways of insulin resistance.

Thus, reversing prediabetes is about controlling blood sugar and insulin levels through *what we eat, what we don't eat, and when we eat* and supporting normal hormone levels through physical movement, sleep, and lowering stress. That's it! Because there are no products to buy, building insulin sensitivity (i.e. actually reversing prediabetes and diabetes and restoring metabolic health) isn't profitable.

Telling people not to buy the foods and drinks that cause insulin resistance and prediabetes is not profitable. Nobody makes money if people aren't constantly distracted by stuff that doesn't work, yet brings in the profits such as another calorie-counting diet that *will* fail over time. The point is profits, and in order to increase profits people have to be constantly distracted into buying the latest trendy vitamin or supplement, spending money on elaborate meal plans that don't address the fundamental hormonal problem, or distracted into buying expensive exercise equipment, etc. You don't need any of this stuff.

Instead I give you a grocery list of staples from which to make many kinds of meals, a cooking and meal prep guide to save you time, and a discussion of functional exercise that doesn't involve buying workout gear, clothing, or memberships. This book does not contain recipes for 3 reasons: a.) I am an historian of science, not a trained chef; b.) as we'll discuss, the low-carb eating pattern is a *continuum*, and how strict you need to be on this continuum depends on many factors that we'll discuss, so instead c.) I give you the ingredients and staples from which to make many kinds of wonderful, quick, low-carb meals that help you control blood sugar and reverse your insulin resistance so you can choose ingredients and staples based on how low-carb you need to be in order to reverse your level of insulin resistance and prediabetes. In subsequent chapters we'll discuss how to determine your level of carbohydrate tolerance because a low-carb eating pattern is not a one-size-fits-all process.

It's shameful but the culture wants us to focus on buying stuff, including all kinds of diet programs that don't work and can make things worse. Reversing prediabetes should not be expensive, cumbersome, or frustrating. It will take time and consistency, but with realistic expectations and in following the four steps in this book, you can definitely do it.

Based on decades of experience and data, including skyrocketing rates of obesity, diabetes, prediabetes, hypertension, NAFLD, cardiovascular disease and other diet-driven conditions, it's clear that all the calorie-reduction diets we try, low-fat nonsense, and incorrect dietary advice are making things worse. There is only one thing that does work: *removing* the cause of insulin resistance, which is too much dietary carbohydrate, most especially refined grains, flour, and sugar in all forms. *Removing* this root cause, carbohydrate toxicity, is *90% of the battle.*

We also *save* money when we're no longer buying all the foods/drinks driving insulin resistance and prediabetes—especially processed and prepared foods, which are very expensive, and wesave a lot of money by avoiding expensive medications to "manage" conditions and diseases we can actually reverse through diet. As a culture, we also need to move around more, improve our sleep, and do what we can to reduce stress—because doing these things improves insulin sensitivity and therefore blood sugar.

The four steps in this book cost nothing, and they work. The problem is that too many industries, especially the processed food giants, stand to lose *a lot of money* if we do the four simple things that reverse our metabolic health problems, including prediabetes and diabetes.

Many in the medical and nutrition science and health professions still believe the wrong paradigms about diet and metabolic health problems because they've been steeped and trained in them—these narratives are dogma, not science. It's very difficult to go against what you've been taught and practiced for decades—even when the science itself is giving us a very different and very clear picture. It takes time for narratives to catch up to the rigorous science and for paradigms to shift.

Insulin Resistance Drives Excessive Hunger

Keep in mind that if losing weight is something you need to do, becoming insulin sensitive again *is the means* by which to lose weight safely and keep it off—not worrying about calories, which the body doesn't understand at any level. Weight loss is the natural byproduct of having less insulin in the blood, i.e. lower levels of the fat storage hormone. (Remember, when insulin levels are high in the body, your fat stores are locked down.

When you lower your insulin levels through a diet low in carbohydrate, insulin releases the locks so to speak, and your body begins releasing fat. This locking and unlocking process is hormonal, not caloric.) As you lower the amount of sugar and foods that *turn into* sugar (carbohydrate) *and* your cells start getting better at taking up the glucose (sugar) from your blood because your insulin sensitivity is improving, you become less hungry.

When our cells get the energy they need because we're more insulin sensitive, we become less hungry, and sugar no longer piles up in the blood. When you bring down your levels of insulin, which happens when you don't eat a diet that spikes blood glucose, you're *automatically* telling your body to release fat.

There's only one diet that does this: low carbohydrate—most especially a diet that is very low in grains (no matter how "whole grain" they supposedly are), flours, and sugar, both natural and artificial. Remember, unlike carbohydrate dietary fat does not spike either blood sugar or insulin, the storage hormone, which is why *eating fat doesn't make you fat*. Eating above our personal level of carbohydrate tolerance floods the body with sugar—sugar the body has to turn into fat for storage via insulin.

So, in terms of generic medical dietary advice to "cut out carbs," one must quickly determine which carbs to eat, and which carbs to decrease and eliminate. This is a highly individual process because each of us has a different level of carbohydrate tolerance, and that tolerance changes over time and in relation to other factors that we'll discuss, including age, activity levels, sleep, and stress. In terms of the generic advice to watch our intake of "calories," and to "burn" more energy that we consume, these are *entirely beside the point* because weight gain isn't about arithmetic, or a language ("calories") the human body doesn't speak. It's about hormones and how protein, fat, and carbohydrate affect them—along with *when* we eat.

The point is to eliminate all easily digestible carbs, refined carbs, as many sources of sugar as possible, and consume fiber-rich, complex carbohydrates instead. We do this by eating whole foods that the body must *work* to break down. Our bodies are designed through millions of years of evolutionary adaptations to consume foods that exist in nature, not in bags, or packages, or cartons, etc.

This isn't sentimentality or a naïve view of eating, and it's not political; it's how our bodies—all humans—evolved over millions of years. Processed food is *incredibly* recent—less than the blink of an eye in evolutionary terms. The problem lies in the fact that eating unprocessed and whole foods has become politicized, and access to these foods is far too often limited or restricted through multiple mechanisms that *are* political, economic, and social.

Two Sources of Energy: Glucose and Fat

Regarding which carbs to eat and those we should not eat, it's important to know that glucose (sugar) from carbs is one of two ways the human body can get its energy from what we eat. We have another *equally good* source of energy, which is **fat**. (In addition to carbohydrate, the body does convert protein into glucose also, but this is a far less significant source of glucose than carbohydrate.)

Before we discuss foods you should eat and foods that you shouldn't, as well as food timing, exercise, sleep, and stress reduction as the 4 intertwined steps that reverse prediabetes and the insulin resistance causing it, it's important to understand the bigger metabolic picture in terms of these two equally good sources of energy.

These two equally good sources of energy are **glucose** (sugar), primarily from carbohydrate in the diet, and **fat**, both the stored fat in our bodies and the fat we eat. Both glucose and fat provide the human body with energy, but they do so in very different ways metabolically and under different conditions. **You have a choice** as to whether you want to use glucose or fat as your primary source of energy, but we can't use them at the same time. It's one or the other.

This is the most important fact to remember in making this choice between glucose and fat as your source of energy. This book is about using glucose as your primary energy source—but doing so in a way that allows you to reverse the insulin resistance that causes prediabetes.

The reasons the human body is metabolically flexible in terms of being able to use both glucose and fat for energy lies in our evolutionary history. Most of us use glucose (sugar) from carbs for energy. However, if we wish to do so we can also do what humans did for millions of years—our entire evolutionary history—we used fat for energy, both the fat we ate in animal sources and the fat we stored in our bodies.

The human body switches from using glucose to fat as its primary energy source when we remove nearly all the carbohydrate from our diets. Doing this *tells* our bodies to turn to our stored fat and the fat we eat for energy. Diet changes what our bodies use for energy. That's powerful!

During the millions of years of our evolution as a species we didn't need to decide whether or not to eat carbohydrate; carbs were available only intermittently in seasonal fruits and plants depending entirely upon on where people lived. Carbs were either a nonexistent or supplemental component of the human diet for millions of years. We relied very heavily and often exclusively on protein and fat from animal sources; humans *evolved* under these conditions. This is why protein and fat are absolutely essential to all humans for all the work our bodies must do every day such as breathing, immune function, cell maintenance, etc.—all the many, many things our bodies do that we don't consciously control. Carbs are only for energy.

If we don't have any carbs to eat, which is how we lived for the vast majority of our evolutionary history, what happens is that the human liver converts the fat we eat as well as the fat we store in our bodies into something called **ketones**, which are what provide us with energy instead of sugar (glucose) from carbs. We can't burn fat directly, so the liver transforms dietary and stored fat into the ketones that our bodies can use.

The reason human babies are so fat compared to other mammals—i.e. have a lot of fat on their bodies—is because *babies need* a lot of ketones in order to fuel healthy brain development, a process that is very energy-intensive given the size and complexity of the human brain, and babies get these ketones from the fat in their bodies and from breast milk, which is very high in saturated fat. Ketones are incredibly important in order for the human brain to develop; and in many ways the adult human brain actually prefers ketones to glucose although it needs some of the latter, which we'll discuss.

The most important thing to remember is that the human body will only switch from glucose to fat as a source of energy if our glucose levels from the carbs we eat (and to certain degree the protein we eat) *go low enough for long enough*—and if our insulin levels go low enough for long enough. When these two things happen, the human body turns to its "backup generator" of energy, fat. We *tell* the body to do this via the ketogenic or "keto" diet on which we consume very little carbohydrate, a moderate amount of protein (to keep glucose levels low), and a *high level of fat*—up to 75% of our diet.

This diet mimics the *metabolic* state of starvation—*without the actual starvation*—so our bodies automatically switch from relying on glucose to relying on fat for energy, fat that the liver converts into the ketones our bodies use for energy, including the brain.

As the most strict end of the of a low-carb diet continuum, the ketogenic diet *tells* the body, at the metabolic level, to use fat (ketones) instead of glucose for energy. The diet itself *changes* what your body uses for energy. As we discussed earlier in this *Introduction*, diet is incredibly powerful. This ability to use diet (the ketogenic diet) to change the very nature of how the human body obtains and uses energy shows us the enormous power we have in choosing what to eat and when to eat.

The keto diet originated as a medical diet to stop epileptic seizures, which it does. It's a very powerful diet with very powerful metabolic effects including effects on the brain; if you take any medications or have any medical condition, it's important to work with healthcare providers who are knowledgeable about how the keto diet works at the metabolic level. Your medications may need to be adjusted—and you can run the risk of hypoglycemia if you're on any medication to lower your blood sugar. If you have cardiovascular disease or any heart problem, you must be especially careful of possible hypoglycemia.

Yet, it's not necessary (or advisable) for everyone with prediabetes to go on the keto or ketogenic diet. It's a medical diet that puts the human body into a different metabolic state. It's also not a fad—it's the diet humans ate for the vast majority of our evolutionary history—we just didn't understand until recently *how* our bodies worked if we removed the toxic levels of carbohydrate that have dominated our diet for just a few decades. Now we do understand. Again, keto isn't the right diet for everyone, but there is also significant resistance in the medical and dietary worlds to the low-carbohydrate continuum in general, *which is not based on robust science*. It's based on ideology, the threat to corporate profits, entrenched ideologies, fear of losing research funding, dietary and medical dogma, and other factors.

Thus, low-carb and keto eating patterns are often discussed as fads in the *narratives* of nutrition science and medical advice—but not because they are fads. Eating below your carbohydrate tolerance is the most powerful and effective way to reverse chronic metabolic diseases, including prediabetes and diabetes, but it poses a significant threat to many entities. The profits of the *entire* processed food industry, much of our agribusiness economy, and a significant percentage of the pharmaceutical industry depend on us eating carbohydrate to toxic levels. The threat to these profits are the reason low-carb and ketogenic options are dismissed or seen as unhealthy—despite the fact that low-carb *is* the diet of our entire evolutionary history as a species—millions of years.

We don't need any more evidence that excessive carbohydrate consumption is normal given the rates of obesity, diabetes, prediabetes, NAFLD, cardiovascular disease, etc. Instead of addressing the real problem driving insulin resistance, carbohydrate, for economic and ideological reasons we're still being told to do the wrong things such as avoid natural sources of fat, avoid meat, eat huge amounts of carbs and consume light machine oils ("vegetable" oils.) As we've discussed, carbohydrate is not essential for health or survival. It is optional, not required in the human diet, but fat is.

This is our evolutionary history. When we follow the standard advice about calories, and carbs, and "willpower," we fail to lose weight and keep it off, and we can't reverse prediabetes. This bad advice means we're still standing on the tennis court trying to win against the machine firing tennis balls at us. We're not going to prevail.

To take another analogy, if we had to buy car after car after car because each one failed quickly and caused us to get into accidents because of mechanical problems, we would know something was very wrong with both the cars and the manufacturers. If it happened with different makes and models, one after the other, we would understand there was a widespread problem. We would understand that it was an industry-wide problem. We would not blame ourselves.

Yet, with each failure to lose weight and keep it off, control hypertension, reverse prediabetes, reverse cholesterol problems—we're encouraged both directly and tacitly to blame ourselves. Inevitably we're told to reduce calories more, eat far fewer animal products, eat more "whole grains" and carbs, consume more "vegetable" oils, and all the rest of it—i.e. we're told to do *more* of the things that cause these metabolic problems in the first place. Buying another faulty car isn't the answer—fixing the industry is the answer. Similarly, following faulty dietary advice even more rigorously isn't the answer; fixing the bad nutritional and dietary advice itself is the answer, but that's going to take time in terms of how institutions work.

Evolutionary history is very powerful evidence; unfortunately it's not used to help us understand nutrition, diet, diabetes, weight, or other areas of our health. The human body and nature itself always exceed our understanding of them; this is the history of science itself throughout the centuries. It makes no sense to ignore millions of years of our evolutionary history and our physiology so we can keep using the circular logic characteristic of so much nutrition science—much of which is funded by corporations that are heavily invested in the foods and agribusiness products that make us sick—and the corporations that make the medications to "manage" these diet-driven conditions.

The Low-Carb Continuum, Glucose, and Fat

To return to the low-carb diet as a continuum of choices: the keto diet, which is not a fad from the perspective of evolutionary history, is also not your only low-carb option to reverse your prediabetes. Other types of low-carb eating that we'll discuss will let you control your blood sugar and reverse insulin resistance while still using glucose as your primary source of energy. This book is about doing just that.

The keto diet is definitely the right diet for some people either temporarily or for long periods, but it's not right everyone for any number of reasons including its strictness, so it's important to understand how it works and to talk with your doctors before trying it—most especially if you take any medications or have any medical conditions. What's important to understand is that keto and the low-carb eating continuum in general are not recent inventions; this way of eating *is* the dietary history of humans.

As we'll discuss, if the keto diet, the most strict end of the low-carb continuum, is not the best choice for you, there are many changes you can make that will also reverse your insulin resistance, most especially if you make the dietary changes addressed in this book in conjunction with moderate exercise, appropriate sleep, and as much stress reduction as possible because each affects blood sugar. As we discussed earlier in this *Introduction*, the ratio of protein, carbohydrate, and fat in what we eat and drink matters enormously—as does when we eat.

We don't tend to overeat protein; we have an innate sense of how much to consume. The same is true of fat. However, we've been told for decades that fat makes us fat and gives us heart disease, especially saturated fat. It's important to understand why these two things are absolutely wrong because these incorrect beliefs have driven us, as a population, to eat carbohydrate to toxic levels—causing widespread blood sugar problems, insulin resistance, and cardiovascular disease. In order to control intake of carbohydrate, we must understand the importance of natural sources of fat in our diet because fat is one of the two *essential* macronutrients along with protein.

Humans evolved in many different environments all over the planet, and carbohydrate was not a common part of our diet until very, very recently. As a species we survived all over the planet in extraordinarily different physical environments because carbohydrate *wasn't* necessary (essential) to health or survival. If it were, we would have had an entirely different evolutionary history as a species if carbohydrate were necessary either for human survival or human health.

To return to the keto diet itself, which is one option on the low-carb continuum, if a person is in nutritional ketosis, which is when the body is using ketones for energy, which the liver makes from fat, the brain still needs glucose, which the liver also manufactures via something called the gluconeogenesis metabolic pathway. No matter which source of energy we use, glucose or ketones from fat, the brain consumes up to 25% of our daily energy needs, more than any other organ, and it does need glucose. Fortunately, *we make our own glucose* via the liver. If we did not, we would die very quickly.

Thus, we do not need to consume any carbohydrate in the diet in order to get the glucose our bodies need; the human body makes what it needs. (If you take any medication that inhibits gluconeogenesis, you must speak with your doctor before lowering your intake of carbohydrate as you may need to adjust your medications.) Among many functions, the brain needs all this energy to help neurons or nerve cells "fire" or to send signals and to do cell-health maintenance.

Thus, evolutionary adaptations have ensured that we always have a source of glucose for our brains—even if we don't eat any carbohydrate at all, which was most often the case during the millions of years of our evolution as a species. As a species we spent millions of years consuming very fatty animals, i.e. protein and fat. Carbohydrate *was not* the center of our diets when the vast majority of our genes were established over millions of years, so our bodies consider carbohydrate to be *optional*. However, both protein and fat are essential; we die without them.

Carbohydrate is for energy—only energy—but we can also use fat just as easily for energy as well. This metabolic flexibility ensured our survival—and it still does today. We have a choice, but we can't tap into this source of energy, fat, when our insulin levels are high because high insulin, as we've discussed, acts like a lock preventing release of fat from our cells. The only way to turn on our metabolic backup generator of energy so to speak—to use fat (ketones) instead of glucose for energy—is if our glucose and insulin levels go low enough for long enough.

Our bodies use glucose *then* fat, in that order. Our liver continues to make glucose no matter which source of energy we're using. It makes perfect sense that the human body uses glucose from carbs first because the body cannot store carbohydrate, but it *can* store fat. If glucose from carbs were available because we had access to *occasional* sources carbohydrate such as seasonal plants, and the vast majority of plants are toxic to humans, seasonal fruits, occasional sources of honey, tubers, etc. the body will use this glucose from carbs *before* depleting its stores of fat for energy.

Because these sources of dietary carbohydrate weren't constant, humans evolved so that we don't have to rely on the glucose from them; we make our own glucose no matter what, and we used fat (ketones) from much more available animal sources for our energy needs.

The Human Body Resists Weight Loss for Evolutionary Reasons

This metabolic flexibility means that from an evolutionary perspective the human body is also designed to *preserve* fat, not lose it. The human body understands fat as its most important source of energy and survival—because it was—for millions of years. This is the major reason losing weight *and keeping it off* is so very difficult.

Our bodies are designed to *resist* weight loss, and the human body evolved to do everything possible in order to gain it back—most especially by slowing our metabolism in response to calorie-counting diets, which the body *interprets* as famine.

It's not actual famine, but the body doesn't know that. Metabolically the body *understands* a sudden loss of essential protein, essential fat, and quantity of food containing them as starvation and responds accordingly to try and save us. This makes perfect sense from an evolutionary perspective. However, the body does not interpret loss of carbohydrate in the diet as starvation because the body can turn to its fat stores for energy—if our blood sugar and insulin levels are low enough.

When the body perceives that we're experiencing a famine because we're suddenly eating far less, especially much less fat and protein in sources such as fatty meat, which we're constantly told to avoid, our metabolism slows down so we expend less energy—i.e. so we can survive longer under what the body *understands* as famine conditions. (We survived under very harsh conditions and in all kinds of weather outdoors because we ate what the human body must have: protein and fat.)

Remember all those fat babies; fat is *essential* to the development, growth, and survival of the human species. Fat is incredibly important to us: carbohydrates are not important. They are an option; carbs are not what our bodies must have. When we eat a lot of carbohydrate day after day, our bodies turn all that excess glucose into fat for storage.

Thus, when we limit fat in particular but increase sugar (carbohydrate) in "whole grains," processed foods, low-calorie, low-fat foods, juices, etc., the body understands this loss of protein, and especially this loss of fat, in evolutionary terms—not in terms of nonsense such as the *Dietary Guidelines for Americans*[6] (DGA) that are replicated throughout the world—with devastating consequences.

So much nutritional and dietary advice is not based on robust science, let alone millions of years of evolution, or on how the human body actually works. Instead, so much of nutrition "science" is based on drivel such as food frequency questionnaires—which are *not* evidence or data in any recognizable scientific sense. Each iteration of the DGA repeats dogma about saturated fat and carbohydrate. Think of it this way; finding yet another recipe in a Medieval manuscript for turning lead into gold isn't going to prove, once and for all, that alchemy actually exists anymore than doubling down on unproven beliefs and hypotheses, especially about saturated fat and carbohydrates, isn't going to make the DGA accurate or scientific.

Nutritional science studies tell us different things every day—e.g. eggs are good one day/eggs are bad the next, etc.; these are basically the bloatware of scientific publications—quick and easy to churn out and very misleading. These types of studies are extremely common in nutritional science, and when the conclusions of these studies are examined through rigorous methods, they prove to be incorrect 80%-100% of the time. (Remember the analogy of those cars that always breakdown and cause crashes—this is the nutritional science equivalent of an industry-wide problem.)

Thus, although we're told eat a low-fat, high carb diet with plenty of "whole grains," when we lower our intake of fat and protein, *we're telling our bodies* that we're experiencing a famine. This is what

---

[6] U.S. Department of Agriculture and U.S. Department of Health and Human Services. Dietary Guidelines for Americans, 2020-2025. 9th Edition. December 2020. Available at DietaryGuidelines.gov

avoiding these foods *tells* the body in the language it actually understands.

Unfortunately we're still hearing outdated narratives such as "low-fat" means "good," meat and saturated fat mean "bad," etc. The body understands "low fat" and lack of animal products as a threat to survival. When we compensate for the loss of fat by eating more carbs, we *create* the conditions for insulin resistance and diabetes by sending our blood sugar and insulin levels on a rollercoaster each and every day. These are the dietary conditions we've been told are good for us; they're not.

The body *prefers* animal sources of protein and fat because that's our evolutionary history. Our bodies are better at absorbing what we need nutritionally from animal products than from plants—it's just how we are as a species due to our long evolutionary history. Thus, vegetarians and vegans have to be *especially careful* to supplement carefully in order to address nutritional deficiencies, choose their carbs very wisely, and use food timing, exercise, sleep and stress reduction to control blood sugar and insulin spikes.

When we tell our bodies that we're experiencing a famine by cutting off foods such as meat, fat (including saturated fat), nuts and seeds with fat and protein, etc., the body responds by doing *whatever it can* to slow our use of energy in order to help us survive—because it isn't getting the fat (and protein) it needs in a wide range of animal sources of fat such as meat, fish, butter, lard, etc. as well as *natural sources* of plant fat such as olives, avocados, coconut, etc.,—not "vegetable" oils we're told to consume that are made with huge amounts of chemicals and created through intensive industrial processes.

These oils are about as "plant-based" as saying cars are "plant-based" because the plastic and metal materials in them began their existence as raw resources we then transformed through intensive industrial and chemical processes.

Thus, diets and eating patterns that tell us to avoid natural fat and eat more carbs cause the body to believe it's experiencing famine—but *without* turning on its backup source of energy, which is fat. We're still getting enough carbohydrate (i.e. sugar) on a low fat, high-carbohydrate eating pattern to *prevent* the body from turning to fat for energy.

This is the reason the keto diet doesn't slow metabolism like calorie-counting/low-fat diets do and why people feel less hungry on the keto diet. The body *is* getting enough energy *through fat in the diet* and *by turning to stored fat in the body for energy*. But glucose and insulin levels must go low enough for long enough in order for the body to turn on this capacity to burn fat (by converting it into ketones).

Counting calories, removing fat from our diets, and eating more carbohydrate means that high insulin levels are going to continue locking down our fat stores and driving high blood sugar. We're going to gain weight, and our blood sugar is going to keep getting worse. This is the crucial difference between a low-carbohydrate/higher fat diet and any calorie-reduction/low-fat diet. The difference is *metabolic* and *hormonal*, not caloric.

If we lower our intake of dietary carbohydrate, starting with processed and refined carbs and especially sugar, but not to the point of going into nutritional ketosis, *we're still going to get significant benefits* in relation to blood sugar, blood pressure, weight loss, and improvement in insulin sensitivity. Thus, the keto diet is one low-carb option on the continuum, but it's not the only option. You have choices, and we'll discuss these so you can determine how to eat below your personal threshold of carbohydrate tolerance, bring down your blood sugar, and stabilize your insulin levels.

To return to weight loss for a moment, it's very important to understand that the failure to lose weight and keep it off on calorie-counting/low-fat diets *is due to evolution*. This metabolic ability to evade weight loss meant our very survival as a species for millions of years. For nearly all of our history as a species our ability to become *temporarily* insulin resistant and store fat easily from the occasional carbs we ate was a *huge survival advantage*.

However, in our current food environments in which we are absolutely flooded with cheap carbs that turn into *huge* amounts of sugar in the blood very quickly, we end up storing all this excess glucose as fat, because that's what the human body does—and driving our blood sugar higher.

We no longer experience *temporary* insulin resistance in response to seasonal, limited carbs—temporary insulin resistance that let us build up our fat stores to help ensure our survival; we're becoming permanently insulin resistant as a population and jeopardizing our survival through diseases such as prediabetes and diabetes. As insulin resistance and hyperinsulinemia worsen throughout the body, as well as locally in our organs such as the liver and pancreas, we suddenly go from prediabetic to diabetic.

If we're not exercising for *hours* a day, all this excess sugar from a diet high in carbs, especially sugar and refined grains/flours, isn't going to get pushed into our muscles to be used. Eventually our cells stop paying attention when the hormone insulin tries to push more sugar into them—and because the cells are already full of sugar. When our cells no longer pay attention to the hormone insulin, we become insulin resistant—some people mildly so and some people severely so. This process can take years or even decades.

So there are two problems: our cells are insulin resistant *and* they're already full of glucose (sugar) so our insulin levels remain high, which is called hyperinsulinemia. Technically these are two different conditions, but the evidence strongly indicates that insulin resistance leads to hyperinsulinemia. When we have both conditions, insulin resistance and hyperinsulinemia, we're in very serious trouble metabolically. By focusing on rebuilding your insulin sensitivity through the four steps in this book, you will automatically lower the level of circulating insulin and your cells can and will accept and use glucose far better—reversing both problems.

In other words, the four steps that are the subject of this book will address both insulin resistance and hyperinsulinemia. Both are caused by too much carbohydrate, especially easily digestible carbs, as well as sugar in all forms—including all artificial sweeteners and most "alternative" sweeteners. With either insulin resistance or hyperinsulinemia, sugar begins to pile up in the blood. This process accelerates as we move from prediabetes to diabetes—i.e. often we have prediabetes for a period of time, but then there's a *sudden* jump to diabetes. This book will help you reverse this entire Type 2 diabetes process by reversing both insulin resistance and hyperinsulinemia.

Therefore, one of our most important survival advantages, our capacity to store fat via the hormone insulin—i.e. *periodic* insulin resistance in response to occasional sources of carbs such as seasonal berries or honey—has become a serious liability only in the last few decades—for the simple reason that our diet *is far too high in carbohydrate*, especially sugar in many forms, both natural and artificial.

Thus we keep storing more and more fat, and our blood sugar keeps rising higher because we just can't use all that glucose because we don't need that much energy given how we live our lives in a modern context. Our blood pressure responds by getting worse—in response to both higher blood sugar and weight gain. Our triglycerides get worse because triglycerides are a direct measurement of carbohydrate in the diet. These triglycerides that our bodies make are the dangerous type of fat—*not* saturated fat in the diet such as cheese, fatty meat, butter, etc., or LDL cholesterol (which is the myth).

We simply do not need huge amounts of glucose in our bodies; that's a very dangerous **myth**. We need about one teaspoon in our blood for our needs. *One piece* of refined white break turns into about *10-12 teaspoons of sugar* in our bodies, which our bodies must store as fat—while driving up our triglycerides and blood sugar and blood pressure and insulin levels. This inundation of carbohydrate day after day overwhelms the body—which is what's happening to us as a population—all across the globe.

As humans, we cannot store carbohydrate directly, so after all this carbohydrate turns into sugar, our bodies store that sugar as fat for later. Our bodies will use this fat for energy *only* if our glucose and insulin levels *are low enough for long enough*. Fat is like a savings account for the body that it won't use unless it has to; when our glucose levels and insulin levels go low enough for long enough, the body knows it's time to take some funds out of our savings—i.e. start using the fat we've stored as well as the fat we eat.

Counting calories *never* tells the body it's time to take out some saving (start using/releasing fat), and lowering intake of fat never tells the body to start "burning" or using fat for energy. Having low levels of circulating insulin tells our bodies it's time to withdraw our savings (stored fat).

You may be told that the body "prefers" glucose rather than fat for energy. That's another prominent myth, and it's completely wrong. The body *must use* glucose first, primarily from the carbs we eat, because humans can't store dietary carbohydrate directly. The body "prefers" *both* glucose *and* fat for energy for the simple reason that we use both, but under different metabolic conditions. That's the difference. Logically the body "prefers" both glucose and fat as energy sources because it uses both, and in some ways the body actually prefers the ketones from fat as we saw with human babies.

Therefore, the issue isn't about "preference" for glucose from carbs; it's about the *sequence* in which the human body uses these two different but equal energy courses: glucose *then* fat. Sequence and "preference" are two very different things. The body doesn't use glucose first because it prefers to do so; it does so because we can't store carbohydrate directly, but we can store fat. This is millions of years of evolution and adaptation at work so we can survive if we have very few or no carbs to eat—which was exactly the situation for the vast majority of our history as a species.

Agriculture only began about 10,000 years ago, which is just the blink of an eye in evolutionary time. For millions of years prior to agriculture our diets were mostly animal products, including fish, and an enormous amount of fat. Many of the animals we ate had far higher levels of fat than our modern farm-raised animals. We're made to eat fat, store fat, burn fat, which is why all these carbs, low-fat foods, and tons of sugar in myriad forms are causing a global pandemic of insulin resistance and its downstream diseases, including prediabetes and diabetes.

In summary, we *can* eat carbs, but they are *optional* as far as the human body is concerned. We make our own glucose via the gluconeogenesis pathway, and we can covert stored and dietary fat, via the liver, into ketones to burn for energy once our blood sugar and insulin levels go low enough. We are very well adapted to eating significant amounts of fat and using that fat for energy. What we are not adapted for is sugar and all the foods that turn into sugar such as "whole" grains, flours, natural sugar in any form—let alone all the foods such as cereals, pastries, desserts, pastas, etc. that become sugar incredibly quickly in the human body.

When we developed agriculture about 10,000 years ago we weren't eating highly refined grains and flours as we are today, and we weren't eating those whole grains 10,000 years ago in the amounts we're eating them now. Humans also got a lot of physical movement on a daily basis to keep pushing glucose from those grains into our cells.

The problem now lies in the fact we're being told constantly and *incorrectly* by various dietary and medical authorities that carbohydrate is "necessary" because the body "prefers" it; *both of these things are incorrect*. That's not a matter of conjecture; it's settled science. The reasons we're still being told this incorrect information are due to economic, political, and cultural forces as well as nutritional science dogma, not because the science is actually in question. So, if you're told you must eat carbohydrate, that's just not true. If you're told you need carbs in order to get the glucose your brain needs, that's just not true. We make glucose every day of our lives, as we discussed. For many reasons we're *also* being told that we have to eat *huge amounts* of carbohydrate every day, lots of "whole grains" especially, and refined and processed grains and flours for certain vitamins—which we can get through much less toxic animal sources.

Carbohydrate is an optional macronutrient in the human diet. It is not a necessity for human health and survival like protein and fat. We make our own glucose via the liver every day, and we can also burn fat (use ketones) for energy just as well as glucose. Thus, understanding that carbohydrate is an optional, not necessary, macronutrient makes it much easier to decide which carbs we eat, when we eat them, and why we eat them.

Once we know these facts about carbohydrate that are not open questions scientifically or in relation to how the human body works (e.g. can use glucose or fat, manufactures is own glucose, etc.), we can put aside all the bad nutritional advice—*and there's a lot of it out there*—that we "must" eat huge amounts of carbs, including refined grains and flours and natural sugar in sugary fruits/juices, and that without all these carbs we won't have enough energy—etc. Nonsense! The body relies on protein and fat for the vast majority of our needs.

The point here is that when we understand that carbohydrate is entirely optional in the human diet, but that protein *and* fat are *not optional*, we can prioritize accordingly—and we're far more empowered to ignore all the inaccurate myths and dogma that surround us about carbs and fat in particular. Once we understand that the human body stores the high level of glucose (sugar) from all these carbs as fat, and that all this glucose makes us insulin resistant over time, raises blood pressure, and causes diabetes, the idea that we must flood our bodies with carbohydrate day after day makes no sense at any level.

We're designed through evolutionary processes to become *temporarily* insulin resistant in response to seasonal sources of carbs *as a mechanism for storing fat to be used for energy later*—fat that ensured our survival. We are not designed to be eating carbs all the time at high levels, which results in permanent insulin resistance and ongoing fat storage. Finally, once we understand that eating fat doesn't make us fat or cause heart disease, we have far more freedom to decide which carbohydrates to eat and why as well as to eat the macronutrient we're designed to eat—fat, including saturated fat.

This is not what agribusiness, drug corporations, and processed food/drink companies want. Lowering our intake of carbohydrate, particularly in processed and refined forms, reduces their profits. Given that medical education, nutritional science and research, and many health organizations are often funded by these entities, it's not surprising we're still getting the same incorrect and dangerous advice that's caused the global metabolic health crisis in the first place.

They want us to continue believing we'll fall down with no energy unless we consume carbohydrate to toxic levels including processed and refined grains and flours. Nonsense! We do *not* need all this glucose; it's protein and fat that the body needs for the vast majority of its functions.

Bad nutritional advice has warped our metabolic health priorities for decades by telling us that the one optional macronutrient, carbohydrate, is essential while telling us that fat, which is absolutely necessary for human survival and health, is optional and dangerous. Treating carbohydrate as necessary, including refined and processed grains, and fat as optional and harmful has caused this pandemic of metabolic health problems globally, including prediabetes, diabetes, hypertension, obesity, and cardiovascular disease.

Thus, if you're told that the body "prefers" glucose from carbs, remember that's not factually correct in terms of how the body actually works. The body *must* use this glucose from carbs first simply because the human body developed over millions of years in environments in which fat and protein were plentiful from animal sources, but carbohydrate was far less available or entirely absent due to temperature, soil conditions, water, etc. and the fact that we didn't start engaging in agriculture until incredibly recently in human history.

We're designed to live on animal protein and fat because that's what was plentiful for millions of years as we evolved as a species—and as our genes were established. It makes no sense from an evolutionary perspective that the human body would depend, for its very survival, on a macronutrient (carbohydrate) that was available only intermittently or not at all. This is not how evolution works.

This is why our bodies are having such difficulty coping with the amount of carbohydrate we're eating now—especially in all these highly refined and processed forms such as wheat, rice, corn, including all these supposedly "whole grains," as well as in obvious forms such as soda, desserts, candy, pasta, bread, starchy vegetables, far too much sugary fruit and fruit juices, sodas, etc.

Our chronic, metabolic health problems show us the vast difference between millions of years of evolution and just a few decades of being flooded with cheap carbs and sugar in all kinds of forms, cheap carbs and sugar that are extremely profitable for corporations and the entities they fund. Human physiology is ancient; cheap and constant sources of carbs and myriad sources of sugar in particular are a *very* recent thing.

This is the reason our bodies and our modern, refined, carb-centered diet are so incompatible, and the consequence of this fundamental incompatibility is skyrocketing rates of prediabetes, diabetes, high blood pressure, high triglycerides, which are a direct measurement of the carbs in the diet, nonalcoholic fatty liver disease (NAFLD), cardiovascular disease, and dementia.

Our capacity to use fat for energy and survive without any carbohydrate is how evolutionary processes ensured our survival as a species over millions of years. Protein *and* fat are actually what our bodies *expect* and are best designed to use. If we didn't have this backup generator for energy, the ability take fat and convert it into ketones for our energy needs, we would have gone extinct really quickly as a species because sources of carbohydrate were often not available for weeks or months at a time—if at all. If we couldn't provide the brain with the glucose it needs through gluconeogenesis, we would have gone extinct as a species.

Yet, these things aren't just a matter of ancient history. We don't need to eat any carbs in order to have enough glucose. If we couldn't create our own glucose on daily basis through gluconeogenesis, instead of waking up every morning we would die. Very early each morning the human liver ensures the glucose (sugar) levels in our bloodstream go up so that after sleeping for many hours we *can* wake up; waking up takes a lot of energy, especially for the brain, which means we need more glucose in our blood. The liver makes sure this happens; this is gluconeogenesis at work each and every day. It's the very reason we wake up at all. We don't have to eat in order to wake up; the liver makes the glucose we need in order for us to wake up.

If we choose to use glucose as our source of energy, we need to eat enough carbs—but we can't flood our systems with them day and night, which we've been doing as a population, especially in processed foods that become sugar incredibly quickly. We also need to be incredibly careful about sugar, including fruit and especially juices. We just do not need high levels of carbohydrate in our diet; that is the most damaging health myth that we're told in various ways from medical and dietary authorities.

We're eating *way more* carbs than the body ever needs, or can use, and we're eating them over long periods of the day, so we're becoming insulin resistant and storing all this glucose from these carbs as fat. This is driving up blood sugar, blood pressure, triglycerides, and it's a *major* contributor to heart disease and dementia. When blood sugar stays high the in brain, it kills our brain cells. Insulin can't get into the brain to bring those sugar levels down, so our essentially our brains marinate in sugar.

We're inundating our bodies with glucose, and insulin just can't get all that excess glucose into our cells, so we're becoming extremely insulin resistant as a population and as a species. Insulin resistance is increasing faster globally than diabetes. This means hundreds of millions of people across the globe are insulin resistant—a metabolic pandemic.

The point is that all this dietary carbohydrate, especially sugar and fructose in sources such as high fructose corn syrup in drinks and processed foods, is driving global insulin resistance at breathtaking speed. This is very, very recent in human history. It's an astonishing change in the human species after millions of years when we were not diabetic, not overweight, and not hypertensive as a species. All of this has happened in just a few short decades. These are exactly the decades in which we have put carbohydrate the center of the human diet—with disastrous consequences across the globe.

Thus, the generic medical advice to "cut carbs" in order to reverse prediabetes doesn't get a person very far in addressing the actual problem, which is figuring out your *individual and personal level* of carbohydrate tolerance in relation to both your blood sugar and your specific level of insulin resistance. This is not a one-size-fits-all process.

With regard to carbohydrate, which is what raises blood sugar the most and therefore insulin secretion, this book will help you understand why fiber-filled and micronutrient-rich carbs are a key part of the solution to prediabetes and insulin resistance—if you wish to keep using glucose instead of fat as your source of energy.

Again using either glucose or fat as your primary energy source is fine from nutritional and metabolic perspectives; each has advantages and disadvantages. The primary disadvantage of the keto diet being that it's very strict. Either glucose or fat works for the human body as a fuel source, but we have to eat differently contingent upon which one we choose. What we **cannot** do is eat a diet that's high in *both* carbs and fat.

Remember, if we have high levels of glucose and insulin in our system from those carbs, our bodies *will not release fat*, including our stored fat. We'll just keep storing all that glucose from carbs as fat *and* we'll also store the fat we eat.

This is what happens when we eat high levels of carbs and fat together. If we cut calories—i.e. we cut fat in particular because it's higher in calories—we send our bodies into metabolic *starvation* mode and slow our metabolism, which means we have to eat less and less (and less) in order to avoid gaining weight. Ultimately we damage our metabolism permanently.

When we control our intake of carbohydrate, we lower glucose (sugar) and insulin levels, so we start releasing fat—i.e. we lose weight. Our bodies understand this dietary language of enough fat and enough protein *and far less carbohydrate* as the signal to release fat safely. The body does not perceive this as starvation because it isn't; the body is getting both essential macronutrients, fat and protein. It doesn't miss the carbs because they're optional as far as the body is concerned. The body doesn't think it's experiencing a famine when we eat enough protein and fat, so your metabolism won't slow down to protect you from that perceived famine.

Keep in mind that you have a choice: use glucose or use fat for your energy. The keto diet is the right diet for many people but not necessarily for everyone. Each source of energy, glucose or fat, has different implications metabolically, and there are advantages and disadvantages to each one. You have a choice. The point is that you can still use glucose as your primary source of energy without *overwhelming* the body with it.

We don't keep filling the gas tank after it's full—there's no reason to do so. Just as gas will spill everywhere if we do that, sugar "spills" into the blood if we keep filling our bodies with it—i.e. through far too much carbohydrate that *all* turns into sugar.

If you choose to use glucose from carbs as your primary source of energy instead of using fat, you need to figure out your level of *carbohydrate tolerance*. This means how many carbs you need for your specific energy needs without overloading your system so that excess glucose piles up in the blood as high blood sugar and gets stored as fat and continues to worsen your insulin resistance over time. Remember, we don't need huge amounts of glucose unless we're engaged in huge amounts of strenuous physical exercise or manual labor.

One of the key reasons we get excessively hungry is because we are insulin resistant; we're not getting the energy from all this glucose because the hormone insulin can no longer successfully usher it into our cells to be used for energy; we're insulin resistant and/or our cells are already too full of glucose. When we become *insulin sensitive* again, we are far less hungry because our cells are getting the glucose we need for energy, and it's not piling up in the blood (pre/diabetes).

You can reverse prediabetes without going on the keto diet; keto is definitely one option on the low-carb continuum, but it's not the only option. The point is that you have choices. Low-carb is a continuum—and it's not a fad, neither is keto. Low-carb and keto *are* the dietary history of our species. This is how we ate for millions of years of our evolution.

It's only in the last few decades that we've completely reversed things and started consuming carbs, especially sugar and refined grains and flours, at such levels. Our bodies can't catch up and metabolize all this carbohydrate because they're not designed this way.

In terms of solving the problem of insulin resistance, the primary focus needs to be on diet. Rather than provide you with recipes for low-carb meals, I give you a concise shopping list of essential food staples; these are staples with which to fill your pantry and use in cooking many kinds of cuisines.

You do not need to be a trained chef to make *incredibly* delicious meals that will keep your blood sugar within normal range, trigger your body's satiety hormones so that you do not want to overeat, and help your body regain its insulin sensitivity. This will happen much more quickly if you include exercise/activity, stress reduction, and if you are disciplined about good sleep.

It takes time—sometimes up to 2 decades—for prediabetes and its underlying insulin resistance to develop. It will take time to reverse it, but the *amazing* thing about the human body is that we *can* reverse serious disease processes, including prediabetes, Type 2 diabetes, obesity, hypertension, NAFLD, etc. The human body has an extraordinary capacity to heal—even into very old age—*if we work with it instead of against it.*

The human body has real limits in terms of how much carbohydrate it can tolerate. This is the way we're designed through the millions of years of evolution. Some of us can tolerate more carbohydrate than others; it's just not the same for everyone. Thus, each person's carbohydrate tolerance is different, and that tolerance to carbohydrate lessens with age.

This is why calorie-counting diets are pretty much beside the point; it's not the calories, it's the insulin resistance from years of a high carb diet, especially sugar in all forms, that drives prediabetes and diabetes. Remember, as a species *we're meant* to eat protein and natural sources fat (not "vegetable" oils, which are *not* natural), and carbohydrate is entirely optional provided we consume enough protein *and* fat.

You might even eat more calories in foods such as cheese, olive oil, avocados, and meat, which is fine. Prediabetes and metabolic syndrome itself are diet-driven, hormonal problems. They are *not* problems of arithmetic. The body itself can't add up or subtract calories—because it has no mechanisms for doing so. Our cells and genes and organs can't do arithmetic. This may sound absurd, but that's because the idea of our bodies somehow counting calories in the foods we eat after we eat them is absurd. *We* can count calories; *our bodies can't.*

Thus, to reverse prediabetes, the focus must be on what you eat, when you eat, and especially on what you don't eat, *not on counting calories or calorie restriction*. The calories in/calories out model doesn't work because the human body is *not* an enclosed system that remains constant in terms of energy. Some dietary and medical authorities justify counting calories as the way to control intake and expenditure of energy by referring to concepts of energy in physics or other fields, which doesn't work because the human body responds to foods in *biochemical* ways, not in terms of physics or math. We don't use energy the way machines do, which is why the comparison doesn't work and never did.

In other words while "calories" exist in other fields of science, they do not apply to the human body. We are not a perfectly enclosed system. Our energy needs and expenditures change all the time depending on many factors; we're not furnaces or steam engines. Our hormones, metabolic pathways, genes, cells, organs, etc. are a lot more complex than a simple calculator adding up and subtracting calories every time we eat or drink, and we're not engines burning coal or gas. We are far more complex.

Instead of talking about an idea that comes from the Victorian period, "calories," we must focus on foods that work *with our bodies from an evolutionary* perspective, foods that signal that we're full, and foods that help control blood sugar—in conjunction with appropriate amounts of physical movement and adequate sleep in particular. Those foods are primarily protein and fat followed by controlled intake of optional carbohydrate in natural sources.

Appetite, Metabolism, and Fat

If you eat the right things in the right combinations (both macro- and micronutrients), your body will tell you that you're full. *Our bodies are designed to do this*. This evolutionary fact is the most powerful, consistent, and robust way to control appetite.

All calorie-reduction diets "work" until they don't, which is the vast majority of the time. The problem is that a diet high in carbohydrate, especially refined and processed carbs, also impairs the hormonal signals that tell us when we're hungry and when we're full. For example, the feeling that we can processed foods, desserts, etc. and never feel full is real; we don't feel full because these "foods" circumvent our natural hormonal signals that tell our brain when we're full. We're literally not getting the message in our brains to stop eating.

Because calorie restriction slows metabolism, we begin to gain weight. If we focus on high carbohydrate, "low calorie" foods instead of getting enough fat as well as protein, we're going to drive our blood sugar and insulin levels through the roof—sugar that will all get stored as fat while our metabolism is slowing down. As we've discussed, metabolism slows down on a low calorie diet because our bodies want to get back to our highest weight when they perceive, metabolically, that we're experiencing a famine—especially when we're eating too little natural fat (*not* vegetable oils).

Evolution is responsible for this survival process—i.e. for preserving fat by slowing metabolism. We can't rewrite evolutionary history. Losing weight does improve blood sugar; but counting calories is *not the way* to lose that weight. *Improving insulin sensitivity* by restricting carbs that promote insulin secretion is the way we lose weight without slowing our metabolism.

As we've discussed, preserving fat is a very successful evolutionary adaptation that served us extremely well in ensuring the survival of the human species over millions of years. This advantage is still with us; for example, there is evidence that people who have a few extra pounds have better survival rates when seriously ill than those who are very lean. Our bodies are *designed* to conserve fat, some of us more than others; however, the wrong diet of refined carbs, too much sugar, artificial sweeteners, eating too often and too much has pushed this survival trait into overdrive, which is the problem.

The way to lose weight is to stop eating all the carbs that quickly increase blood sugar and therefore insulin response. Insulin is also the fat storage hormone; so when we have high levels of insulin circulating in response to constant spikes in blood sugar, we're *telling* our bodies to store fat. When we lower our blood sugar by controlling intake of carbs, especially sugar in all forms, we have less circulating insulin—i.e. lower levels of the fat storage hormone. Doing so *tells* our body to start *releasing* fat—i.e. weight loss.

As we've discussed, reversing prediabetes as well as losing weight are all about controlling blood sugar spikes and insulin spikes. It's a hormonal process, not a caloric one. The reason calorie-counting diets don't work is that the human metabolism *resets* itself in response to what it understands as starvation. Your body doesn't know you're on a "diet" and trying to lose weight or control your blood sugar.

Your body understands reduction in calories, most especially reduction in protein *and* fat, as a threat to survival, so your body automatically slows your metabolism, makes you a lot more interested in food, and makes exercise/movement feel more difficult. These are some of the ways in which the body reacts to calorie-counting diets *that lower fat intake and increase carbohydrate intake*, which is typically what calorie-restriction diets do—exactly what we should *not* do if we want to reverse prediabetes, become insulin sensitive again, and control our weight over time.

Both protein *and* fat are **essential** for all of our metabolic functions; carbohydrates are only for energy—and they are one source of energy—fat is the other, *equally good* source of energy. So when we restrict fat and protein as a way of decreasing calories, we're decreasing the two macronutrients that are absolutely critical to *all the things our bodies must do all the time* from breathing, to building and maintaining our bone density, to maintaining our immune system, etc.

Carbohydrates don't provide energy for any of this work, which is the vast majority of the work our bodies must do constantly. It's not carbohydrate but *both protein and fat* that enable our bodies to do this work. Finally, low-calorie diets typically mean we increase easily digestible carbs and dramatically lower fat in particular, which sends our blood sugar and our fat storage hormone insulin through the roof causing us to gain more weight and putting us on track to develop diabetes.

When we replace protein and fat (which are essential) with low-calorie processed foods in particular, we're really harming our bodies —literally starving them. The body reacts for its own survival and slows our metabolism. This is the reason calorie-reduction diets "work" for about 6 months, and then our bodies slow our metabolism so that the number of calories we ate to lose weight *becomes* the amount of calories that now make us *gain* weight. This is why we start gaining the weight back—and more—even if we're still eating the same number of calories.

This is why the math doesn't work in terms of "counting" calories. We aren't failing to "stick" to a diet; our metabolism has changed in response to the threat of starvation—the threat of too little fat in particular. When we eat adequate protein *and* fat, we *don't* starve our bodies, because these (not carbs) are the body's sources of energy for the vast majority of our daily needs.

If you decide you want to try the strictest version of the low-carb diet, the keto diet, there are real benefits as well as drawbacks and potential complications for those with elevated blood sugar and Type 2 diabetes, especially in relation to possible hypoglycemia if you take medications that lower blood sugar. Therefore, it is essential that you work with medical professionals who are well informed about the ketogenic diet before embarking on it.

As you'll see in this book, you can still use glucose as your primary source of energy *and* reverse your insulin resistance and prediabetes.

Keep in mind that both high blood sugar and insulin resistance are also problems that have everything to do with the food options available to us, priorities in the food industry such as transportation and shelving positions, profit margins, etc. Our ancient survival trait to conserve fat—essentially temporary insulin resistance during times when we could get carbs such as tubers, fruit, or honey—has been pushed into constant overdrive because of bad information about carbs, a diet that's simultaneously high in both carbs and fat, and too much snacking, which keeps insulin levels elevated for long periods.

Finally, the history of the diet industry is littered with very profitable fads that ultimately work against our physiology and worsen obesity—so people have to keep trying "new" diets—nearly all of which worsen our weight problems over time as well as other metabolic health problems.

Prediabetes and Insulin Resistance

Let's review the basics of prediabetes and insulin resistance in order to better understand the dietary essentials, exercise, food choices, hormonal signaling, and blood sugar testing outlined in this book.

First, to review the terminology "prediabetes" became a diagnosis only very recently, and technically it's not a disease. In 2010 American Diabetes Association (ADA) determined that "prediabetes" should be used as an umbrella term. Some argue that the epidemic of prediabetes, 80+ million people in the US, 1 out of 3 adults, is actually driven by the pharmaceutical industry, i.e. medicalization of normal bodily functions or processes, and that the "epidemic" of prediabetes scares people unnecessarily.

Yet, when one looks at the actual science of how prediabetes (intermediate hyperglycemia) affects the body, one sees that this is definitely not an empty diagnostic category. It gives us an extremely valuable window of time to make lifestyle changes that robust evidence shows work better than medication to stop a disease that is extremely serious, even in its earliest manifestation of prediabetes. The data is clear on prediabetes; lifestyle changes, especially diet, and exercise, work better than the first-line drug, Metformin. Further, prediabetes means a high risk for developing diabetes with yearly conversion rate of 5%-10% to diabetes, so using this window of opportunity to reverse the diabetes process itself is important.

Over time, that's a serious risk of conversion to diabetes. Even in the prediabetic stage one can get early nephropathy, small fiber neuropathy, early retinopathy and risk of macrovascular disease. Blood sugar in the prediabetes range can increase our risk of cardiovascular disease and dementia. High blood sugar affects all of our organs, including the heart and the brain.

What Causes Prediabetes?

As we've been discussing, the short answer is **insulin resistance**. Prediabetes and diabetes are points on a continuum of high blood sugar. High blood sugar is *one symptom* of the bigger, underlying problem of insulin resistance that has many negative consequences for the body. High blood sugar also means higher levels of inflammation in the body and suppression of the immune system, a higher risk of cardiovascular disease and dementia, and much higher risk of obesity/weight gain and hypertension. Insulin resistance and too much circulating insulin (hyperinsulinemia) drive this cluster of diseases.

Just to review how insulin resistance works, it's when our cells no longer respond properly to the hormone insulin whose job it is to push or usher sugar (glucose) out of the blood and into the cells where it is used as energy. When our cells ignore insulin then the sugar accumulates in the blood, which we call prediabetes then diabetes. Thus, improving insulin sensitivity—the ability of insulin to usher glucose into our cells—is how we control blood sugar over time. Controlling blood sugar is also crucial to lowering systemic inflammation, which underlies so many other disease processes, including most cases of cardiovascular disease and many types of cancer.

In some cases prediabetes can happen because the pancreas doesn't produce enough insulin, which is different from insulin resistance. However, the major reason most people develop prediabetes is because they're insulin resistant due to a diet that's far too high in carbohydrate. This diet also impairs the pancreas by causing it storing too much fat—which happens when our bodies convert glucose into fat. The more glucose in our bodies the more fat we have to store both in our fat cells and in our organs—first in the liver then in the pancreas. Organs such as the liver and the pancreas can then become insulin resistant; so we can have both localized insulin resistance in our organs that impairs them as well as insulin resistance more widely in the body.

High blood sugar (high blood glucose) does a lot of damage at the cellular level, in our organs and in our cells, even when it's well below the official 6.4% A1C test result that marks the threshold of diabetes. "Prediabetes" is diagnosed when the A1C result falls between 5.7-6.4%, but recent studies indicate that 30% of people with prediabetes have retinopathy, and other studies have shown vascular damage in the prediabetic range as well as other problems including heart disease, stiffened arteries and blood vessels, high triglycerides, and high blood pressure. Therefore, prediabetes means there are already real problems going on throughout the body. *So, think in terms of diabetes, not "pre" diabetes.*

Often one sees the triad of high triglycerides, high blood pressure, and high blood sugar together. These don't always show up in test results at the same time, but insulin resistance caused by a diet that's too high in carbohydrate also drives these conditions too. The earliest indication of insulin resistance is often high blood pressure—even when the A1C test is normal. If you have one or more of these conditions, you must address the underlying chain of causation that begins with insulin resistance—caused by consuming a diet that's too high in carbs, especially grains and flours well as sugar in any form, including natural forms such as sugary fruits, as well as artificial sweeteners of any kind.

Body type—the "apple"—with fat around the waistline almost universally correlates with elevated insulin levels. Subcutaneous fat in other parts of the body does not drive insulin resistance in the same way as fat around the waistline does. This is because abdominal adiposity means excess blood glucose is getting stored as fat inside the liver and pancreas, and that means these organs can't function properly. Fat in these organs is part of the process in which prediabetes becomes diabetes.

As insulin resistance worsens, and it's becoming clear that this process can happen over decades, it triggers a series of responses in the body to deal with rising blood sugar, specifically this process of storing high levels of glucose as fat in the liver, pancreas, and abdominal area in particular.

This causes serious problems in these organs. Fructose is especially dangerous for the liver, most especially in forms such as high fructose corn syrup that's common in drinks and processed foods. For example, non-alcoholic fatty liver disease (NAFLD) and Type 2 diabetes (T2DM) regularly co-exist; further, they act synergistically to drive negative outcomes. When someone has both NAFLD and Type 2 diabetes there's an increased likelihood of diabetic complications including both macro- and micro- vascular complications.

The way to reverse non-alcoholic fatty liver disease is to significantly reduce intake of dietary carbohydrate and eliminate fructose, most especially the high fructose corn syrup in drinks and processed foods; it's *incredibly* toxic to the liver, which is the only organ that can process it.

Excess glucose in the blood from a diet high in carbohydrate, especially sugar, also ends up getting stored as fat in the pancreas, which further harms this organ that produces insulin. Fat in the pancreas further diminishes the capacity of insulin to push glucose from the bloodstream into the cells. Given that insulin is also the fat (energy) storage hormone, this state of insulin resistance then prompts the body to store more of this excess blood sugar as fat. All this circulating blood sugar ends up piling up in the blood and finally shows up in an A1C test when it can no longer be cleared from the body or stored as fat in the organs and tissues. As insulin resistance worsens, the body suddenly goes from being prediabetic to diabetic.

So, when glucose starts piling up in the blood, this is the *last stage*, not the first. The underlying insulin resistance driving this process can go on for years before A1C and fasting glucose tests finally start showing elevated blood sugar. It's far quicker to test the blood (A1C and fasting glucose tests) than it is to test the liver and pancreas for stored fat, and unless you ask specifically to be tested for insulin resistance, most MD's are not going to do it, especially if you're in the prediabetic range. In part the reason for this is that if you're prediabetic, your MD already knows you are insulin resistant.

The problem lies in the fact that we're not testing for insulin resistance routinely along with other basic tests like blood pressure, cholesterol, etc. If we tested routinely for insulin resistance, which drives prediabetes and diabetes, we would identify the problem *long before* people developed prediabetes, Type 2 diabetes, hypertension, obesity, most cholesterol problems, NAFLD, and cardiovascular disease. Instead, as a culture we're waiting until these diseases show up downstream from the actual cause: insulin resistance and too much circulating insulin in the body.

Keep in mind that when A1C is in the prediabetic range, there's much more going on metabolically and in terms of damage to the body. A1C results are like the visible part of an iceberg; under the surface of the water the iceberg is much bigger and much more dangerous. That iceberg is insulin resistance.

Type 2 Diabetes is Not a Progressive Disease

There is evidence of a genetic predisposition toward insulin resistance especially in certain populations; however, Type 2 diabetes (and therefore prediabetes) is overwhelmingly a dietary disease worsened by lack of exercise, high levels of stress, and sleep deprivation.

One night of sleep deprivation can drive blood sugar up significantly and impair the immune system; and when one is insulin impaired, which is what a high A1C indicates by measuring one symptom—high blood sugar—sleep deprivation and stress further worsen insulin resistance and blood sugar.

Therefore diabetes (and prediabetes) is a multifactorial disease. One must address *each factor* beginning with the most significant culprit: a diet high in carbohydrate, most especially sugar in any form. We're often told that diabetes is a "progressive" disease that always gets worse. This is not accurate. It's a disease that will worsen if we don't *reverse* the underlying cause: diet-driven insulin resistance.

If we address this underlying cause, Type 2 diabetes doesn't have to progress. Depending on the level of damage to the pancreas as well as other factors, people can reverse Type 2 diabetes or significantly reduce medications[7]—if they reverse the underlying cause. The belief that Type 2 diabetes is inherently "progressive" and always gets worse is predicated on the *assumption* that people *must* eat carbohydrate—and do so beyond their tolerance levels. Eating this way is not inevitable, let alone necessary, but it's been made to seem as though excessive consumption of carbohydrate is normal. It's not.

---

[7] Athinarayanan S.J., Adams R.N., Hallberg S.J., McKenzie A.L., Bhanpuri N.H., Campbell W.W., Volek J.S., (...), McCarter J.P. Long-Term Effects of a Novel Continuous Remote Care Intervention Including Nutritional Ketosis for the Management of Type 2 Diabetes: A 2-Year Non-randomized Clinical Trial. (2019) *Frontiers in Endocrinology*, 10, JUN 2019. https://doi.org/10.3389/fendo.2019.00348

Carbohydrate is the only optional macronutrient, which means it is not inevitable that people must continue eating it, especially at high levels, and therefore worsen their blood sugar. Because it's an optional macronutrient, each person's level of carbohydrate tolerance is individual and complex; it can and does change over time.

For example, as we age our muscles become less efficient at taking up glucose, and the human metabolism also slows. Thus, as we age we tend to drift toward insulin resistance, which means we have to be especially careful to control blood sugar and insulin resistance through diet, exercise, sleep, and stress reduction.

What we share in common is a culture that promotes excessive carbohydrate intake beyond what the human body is designed to consume or need. We know this because the obesity and Type 2 diabetes rates have skyrocketed in tight correlation with the increased consumption of dietary carbs, especially processed and refined carbohydrates, which are actually recommended in the Dietary Guidelines for Americans[8], which were first published in 1980.

Correlation is not causation, but given the epidemic nature of chronic metabolic diseases and conditions in this country, which looks more like a population exposure phenomenon (e.g. cholera), the evidence is clear that a population regularly exposed to large amounts of carbohydrate, especially refined grains, flours, and sugar, develops widespread metabolic diseases and conditions. This exposure-like pattern has been replicated globally as other countries and cultures began to follow the U.S. DGA and consume more refined carbohydrates, processed foods, and sugar.

---

[8] U.S. Department of Agriculture and U.S. Department of Health and Human Services. Dietary Guidelines for Americans, 2020-2025. 9th Edition. December 2020. Available at DietaryGuidelines.gov

Unfortunately, the **DGA for 2020-2025** continues in this same vein; these Guidelines advocate consumption of carbohydrate well beyond the tolerance of most humans, including sugar and refined/processed carbs. This is the diet that's killing us, and the DGA continues to recommend it for "healthy" Americans. 88% of American adults are now metabolically compromised, and we got this way *because we ate according to these Guidelines.*

The DGA aren't based in science; they're based in ideology, corporate interests, agribusiness profits, and a whole raft of special interests. They're not based in any recognized method of scientific review. They're not based in science at all. They're a complete disaster.

Unfortunately, MD's and dieticians have to follow them, which is why we continue to be told that we "need" to eat lots of "whole grains" as well as processed and refined grains and flours and far too much sugar in any form for "nutritional" reasons. Nonsense! These Guidelines are major reason Americans are now suffering from epidemic levels of obesity, diabetes, hypertension, NAFLD, cardiovascular disease, and dementia—diet-driven metabolic conditions and diseases that are increasing not decreasing.

So, while the dangerous, unscientific DGA now exhort us in simplistic terms to "make every bite count," the question is, *count as what*? Every bite of all the carbohydrate the DGA tells us to eat is still going to add up to a diet that's spiking blood sugar, insulin levels, and causing fat storage across the entire population. New DGA, same as the old DGA.

Just as "calories" are based on nineteenth-century technology, the DGA are based on assumptions that are *decades* out of date—and the DGA review committees keep coming up with ever more implausible ways to say they can't find the current, relevant science. *It's their job* to review the robust science in a rigorous way; the law actually says they're supposed to do that. That is definitely not what's happening.

So, start your reversal of prediabetes by *ignoring* the DGA and the advice based on these Guidelines. Begin with the one factor that *determines blood sugar and insulin levels more than any other factor*: a diet that's too high in carbohydrate, which is an entirely optional macronutrient, and most especially sugar in any form. Do you eat processed foods and sugar, including natural sugar such as honey and too much carbohydrate in general? That's the place to start making real changes, and the list of staples in this book will help you do that.

Is lack of exercise also a problem? How much stress are you under? Do you have sleep problems? All four areas are important: a low-carb diet; increased exercise; stress reduction; and sleep improvement. But you must begin by addressing carbohydrate consumption, eliminating processed foods and drinks, and doing all that you can to eliminate all forms of sugar. This is a process, and it will take time, but the results are *worth it*—now and for years to come.

How Insulin Resistance works

Let's take a moment to review insulin resistance because it's what drives prediabetes in the majority of cases—along with hypertension, cholesterol problems, and weight gain. Insulin resistance happens when our powerful hormone insulin can no longer do one of its hundreds of jobs—which is to prompt cells to take up glucose to be used as energy. Consequently, sugar piles up in the blood.

This process works like lock and key; insulin is the hormonal "key" that "unlocks" specific receptors on cells that allow the glucose to get into those cells and become energy for those cells. In the state of insulin resistance, the hormonal insulin "key" no longer fits into these specialized receptors ("locks") on the cells. To use another analogy, insulin "knocks" at the "door" of the cells ready to usher glucose into them. In the state of insulin resistance, the cells no longer "answer" the door.

Consequently, glucose ends up piling up in the blood and gets stored as fat in the liver and pancreas—especially as "belly" fat –abdominal fat—where it smothers the organs. In turn, this stored fat in the pancreas and liver further impair insulin functioning. (There's both localized insulin resistance in specific organs as well as a generalized insulin resistance throughout the body.) Finally all this sugar in the blood is seen via an A1C test/fasting glucose test. Once it finally shows up in the A1C test, this feedback loop is *well established* in the body, and insulin resistance will get worse. The A1C test is essentially a belated test showing one symptom of insulin resistance, high blood sugar, long after insulin resistance has taken hold in the body.

If one is not in nutritional ketosis via the keto diet and burning fat as one's primary fuel source, excessive intake of saturated fat from animal products can further blunt insulin sensitivity—when one is still using glucose as one's primary fuel source. When one is in nutritional ketosis, one typically eats about 75% of one's diet in fat—because it's the body's fuel source once the liver turns fat into ketones.

When excess blood glucose from high dietary carbohydrate intake gets stored as fat in the liver, which is one of the first places it goes if it can't get into the cells due to insulin resistance, your triglycerides rise. Thus, triglycerides are a clear measurement of the level of carbohydrate in your diet. Blood pressure rises because excess glucose circulating in the blood stiffens the vessels in the body, and the excess weight caused by this process makes blood pressure and blood sugar rise further in a vicious circle.

When the hormonal insulin "key" and cellular "locks" no longer fit, which is the state of insulin resistance, the cells of the body also don't get the glucose they need because the glucose can't get into the cells. This increases appetite because we're not getting the energy we need.

Our brains and organs need us to consume some dietary carbohydrate (veggies, fruit, beans, dairy, etc.) if we're not in nutritional ketosis and using ketones as our fuel source. What we do not need for human health is any of the "bad" carbs in processed foods (including bread) and simple sugars that lack nutritional value, fiber, micronutrients, etc. and *cause* high blood sugar and insulin resistance. We don't need much glucose in our bloodstream for adequate energy; we've been told that we need high levels of glucose from carbs—this is simply not true. As a population we're eating *way over our carbohydrate tolerance*—the data show this in skyrocketing levels of obesity, diabetes, nonalcoholic fatty liver disease, etc.

There's a world of difference between eating limited, fiber-rich, low sugar, whole food carbohydrates such as above ground vegetables, and eating a diet filled with grains, cereals, pastas, flours of all kinds, sugary fruit, juices, desserts, etc. that drive blood sugar and insulin way up day after day, month after month, year after year.

Also, our Dietary Guidelines for Americans (DGA), advertising, and dietary advice since the mid-1980's *lump good and bad carbs together*, which is a major problem. MD's have to use these guidelines ("standard of care"), so their hands are tied in many cases. Dieticians also have to use the DGA as well. The DGA and most dietary advice lumps carbohydrates together that have no business being lumped together given how very differently they affect blood sugar, insulin levels, and fat storage.

Pasta, breads, cereals, refined flours and grains, sugar/fructose, most fruits, juice, etc. are *far worse* for your blood sugar and promote insulin resistance over time; veggies that grow above ground are also carbohydrates, but these don't destroy your blood sugar and cause insulin resistance over time. Beans are unique carbohydrates because they have a lot of fiber, and they have protein, so they don't turn into glucose as quickly as grains, flours, pastas, sugar, etc., but they're also starchy.

This means you determine how foods and drinks affect you individually by testing your blood sugar regularly in response to what you eat. Testing your blood sugar consistently in relation to what you eat and drink, your exercise, sleep and stress will tell you your level of carbohydrate tolerance.

Fruits such as berries, avocadoes, lemons, limes and tomatoes are not nearly as damaging to blood sugar as more sugary fruits. Keep in mind that our cultivated fruits are far sweeter, i.e. contain more sugar, than their wild counterparts, so we're getting more sugar in fruits now than when we ate them during our evolutionary history.

The fact is we do *not* need to eat any refined/processed carbs. (Technically, we don't actually need to eat *any* carbohydrate at all provided that we eat adequate fat and protein. This is because carbohydrate is not an essential macronutrient the way protein and fat are, and the human liver will make the glucose the body needs as we've discussed.) So, eating the *whole food sources* of the macro- and micronutrients we need for human health gets us around the problem of these dangerous Dietary Guidelines for Americans and the horrible advice to eat refined/processed carbs as well as far too much carbohydrate and sugar. In particular processed foods companies *rely* on these Dietary Guidelines for Americans exhorting us to eat lots of carbs, including refined grains and flours, in order to maintain and increase their profits—generation after generation. The same goes with companies that make drinks that spike blood sugar and insulin levels.

The DGA are going to keep promoting "whole grains" and other processed foods as part of a "healthy" diet as we see with the 2020-2025 DGA. Until these Guidelines change to reflect how humans *actually* metabolize food and the causal relationship between carbohydrate (especially refined carbs) and epidemic levels of metabolic diseases and conditions, we're going to continue to be told to eat refined carbs as well as too much carbohydrate in general—and sugar. This advice *is all about making profits*, not human health.

As we've been discussing, humans simply aren't adapted from an evolutionary perspective to eat refined/processed carbs and high levels of sugar/fructose. We are especially not adapted to eating high levels of carbs and natural sugars all year long or for long periods during the day and night. From an evolutionary perspective, we're designed to give our bodies a rest from eating and drinking for periods of time every day. This is how our bodies work, so snacking is a serious problem because it causes our blood sugar and insulin levels to stay high for long periods—contributing to the development and worsening of insulin resistance over time.

Keep in mind that our modern foods are also very different from their wild counterparts, both plants and animals. Fruits are seasonal so we didn't have access to them all year long, and in their wild forms fruits don't contain nearly as much sugar as our cultivated varieties. Honey is also seasonal. Wild animals we hunted for millions of years had *much higher levels of fat*, including saturated fat. The problem now is that we no longer eat seasonally or for limited periods during the day. These two things may seem trivial, but from metabolic and evolutionary perspectives, they're very big contributors to epidemic levels of pre/diabetes, obesity, hypertension and other metabolic diseases and conditions, including cardiovascular disease, which is basically diabetes of the heart.

Our bodies can't properly handle refined carbs such as grains and flours and high levels of sugar/fructose for the very simple reason that processed/refined food *doesn't exist in nature*, and simple sugars are rare (e.g. honey), seasonal, and limited in variety. It's really important to remember that most of our genes were established long before we started to cultivate grains, which was only about 10,000 years ago. This severe disconnect between how our bodies evolved over millions of years and our modern foods and food environments is the crux of the problem.

Telling people they have to stick to a calorie-counting diet is not only wrong because we have no receptors for calories and the body is not an enclosed system of energy like an engine, it's cruel because it does not work, and it makes our health problems much worse. Weight loss is not about willpower; it's about insulin resistance, which is what's *causing* one to eat too much for reasons we've discussed. Address insulin resistance, and appetite normalizes. It takes time, but that's how it works.

In addition to the nonsense about counting calories, unfortunately human health is no longer the priority in the culture. The priorities are corporate profits, ideological biases, transportation needs, shelving priorities, agribusiness demands, politics, funding for nutritional research and advocacy groups, etc. We *can't retrofit* our bodies or change our evolutionary history to suit the needs of the modern processed food industries, agribusiness, drug companies, etc.—the results are chronic, metabolic diseases and conditions, including cardiovascular disease.

Among other things, all this sugar in our bodies from excessive carbs, including too much fruit and juice, promotes high levels of inflammation—most especially refined sugar (including processed foods), and our bodies didn't evolve to consume any of these things in the amount *and* the frequency we do now. In particular, refined sugar suppresses the immune system. It's much better to eat an apple than a candy bar, but if you have any metabolic condition or disease, you may have to limit or eliminate fruit until your blood sugar and insulin levels have improved. As we've discussed, diet is the only way to change the cellular pathways involved in insulin resistance; there is no drug that can do this.

Yet, in our society both refined/processed foods are abundant because they're cheap, easy to chew and swallow, and taste good—especially with all the added salt, sugar, cheap oils, etc. They do not fill the stomach the way real food does, especially in terms of nutritional density. The stomach *knows the difference* between refined junk, and real whole foods, and it sends signals to the brain accordingly. Processed foods lack the density of whole foods, so our brains do not get the hormonal signals from our stomachs that we're full.

This is the reason we can eat huge amounts of processed and refined foods, starches, flours, sugars, and grains; our brains are literally not getting the message (hormonal signals) that we're full. When we eat unrefined, whole, fiber-rich foods, natural fat, and animal products such as meat and fish, our brains absolutely do get the hormonal signals that we're full. Processed food industries know this, which is why processed foods are so profitable—*they target our evolutionary vulnerabilities* so we don't know we're full and will keep eating them.

Refined and processed substances (they're not food!) are plentiful because they're cheap for companies to make and they store easily for long periods of time in stores. Ingredients are cheap, and the profit margins much higher for companies that make them. This "food" is all about manufacturing and distribution needs as well as profits, not the nutritional needs and actual metabolic processes of the human body. We are inundating ourselves with "foods" our bodies weren't designed to handle most especially not in the quantities or frequency we eat them as a society.

All this excess blood glucose from the standard American diet, 60% of which is processed, has to go somewhere, so it gets stored in the liver, pancreas, adipose tissue of the body, etc., and then it begins pooling up in the blood because it has no where else to go. When fat cells become enlarged and therefore distended (misshapen) from storing fat, their receptors become less sensitive to insulin, and those fat cells produce hormones that make the body even more resistant to insulin. Finally, high levels of circulating insulin actually prevent our brains from getting the hormonal signal that we're full—so we keep eating and driving our blood sugar and insulin levels up further.

This process of insulin resistance is a feedback loop. All this carbohydrate turns into sugar in the human body and pools up as high blood glucose and then gets stored as fat in the organs, and the liver releases higher and higher levels of triglycerides. This entire process drives up blood pressure as well, but at the same time, the glucose in the blood is not getting into the cells for energy. Exercise is what helps the insulin do its job and get the glucose into the cells; so combine high blood glucose with our increasingly sedentary and sleep-deprived culture, and it's a perfect storm of insulin resistance and metabolic health problems—the glucose crisis.

Studies are very clear at this point that diet and exercise are actually better and more effective than diabetes drugs to treat "prediabetes." If diabetes were a "progressive" disease, logically it wouldn't improve with diet and/or exercise or other lifestyle interventions because it will always worsen. But as the science clearly demonstrates, "prediabetes" and many cases of Type 2 diabetes are absolutely reversible.

Food Cravings, Insulin Resistance, and Weight Gain

Insulin resistance is what actually drives food cravings, especially for simple carbs like bread, potatoes, rice, corn, and simple sugars, etc. *Insulin resistance is what drives the sensation of being constantly hungry*. High insulin does a couple of things: 1.) prevents our brains from understanding that we're full and 2.) drives us to eat more in the attempt to get glucose into the cells. The hunger is real because glucose is isn't getting into the cells where it's needed for energy; instead, the vast majority of the glucose from a high dietary carbohydrate gets stored as fat (via insulin).

Insulin resistance is especially cruel because it causes us to eat precisely those foods that *worsen* insulin resistance, processed foods and simple carbs, sugar in many forms, all in the attempt to push glucose (energy) into the cells. Recent work in neuroscience shows us that a diet high in sugar, including natural sugar such as juice and fruit, and refined dietary carbohydrate is **very addictive**. Thus, *these cravings are real* as are symptoms of this worsening feedback loop of insulin resistance in which we eat more food, more carbs, and more sugar all in the unsuccessful attempt to get energy (glucose) into the cells. As this cycle continues, the body becomes more and more resistant to letting the glucose into the cells. We also get used to having high blood sugar, and when our blood sugar drops, we crave these foods to raise it. We experience blood sugar swings, mood swings, and we feel "hangry," etc.

So, one must address the actual root cause of high blood sugar: insulin resistance. The *byproducts* restoring your insulin sensitivity through a low-carb diet supported by enough activity /movement/ exercise, adequate sleep, and stress reduction include:

1.) weight loss
2.) decreased food (carb/sugar) cravings
3.) lower blood sugar
4.) lower blood pressure
5.) lower triglycerides
6.) decreased fat in the liver and pancreas and elsewhere

7.) better vascular health
8.) better heart health
9.) better brain health
10.) better immune health.

There are many other "byproducts" of controlling your blood sugar and your insulin secretion, which include not developing Type 2 diabetes and its terrible consequences. Items 1-10 above will improve, maybe not in a linear way or all at the same time, but the science is clear that insulin resistance and high blood sugar drive a vast and complex set of problems in the body.

Prediabetes is Diabetes

As we've been discussing, insulin resistance is a diet-driven hormonal problem, and improving insulin sensitivity by restricting intake of carbohydrate, most especially sugar, *is the key* to addressing multiple metabolic health problems at the same time, including high blood sugar and blood pressure, high triglycerides, chronic inflammation, and fatty liver disease. This process of worsening metabolic health can take years while the body is still doing its best to try and clear the excess sugar (glucose) from the blood as insulin becomes less and less effective in doing so (insulin resistance).

An A1C test can look normal for up to 20 years (!) while insulin resistance worsens along with its multiple health complications throughout the body. These metabolic health problems are the main cause of cardiovascular disease and dementia as well.

So, when you limit your intake of carbohydrate, especially sugar in all forms, you're doing *one thing* that results in *multiple* benefits. When you add more exercise, better sleep, and stress reduction you accelerate this process.

As we've seen, the ability of the body to deal with high blood glucose by storing it as fat eventually comes to an end, and blood sugar begins to rise (and rise). The inevitable weight gain also means hormonally active and distorted fat cells pump out hormones that make this feedback loop worse. Along with weight gain, blood pressure and high triglycerides can show up before the A1C test finally shows prediabetes or diabetes. This is because a diet high in carbohydrate, especially "whole grains," and sugar from both processed foods and natural sources such as fruit and juice, is already getting stored as fat, worsening our blood pressure and driving our triglycerides up.

This process can go on for months or years before sugar eventually pools up in the blood, and we're diagnosed with prediabetes or diabetes. Essentially the A1C test is an indirect measurement of increasing insulin resistance over time.

Tests for insulin resistance do exist, but MD's rarely use them. Insulin resistance is still primarily a subject of research not clinical practice. That is a very serious problem. If we were evaluated routinely for insulin resistance along with blood pressure and cholesterol and weight, we would see this fundamental problem driving so many diseases and conditions much sooner across the population.

Data suggest that 85% of American adults are insulin resistant. We don't know for sure because we're not testing. If we tested routinely for insulin resistance, people could use dietary changes to completely alter the trajectory of their insulin resistance—i.e. *before* all this sugar piles up in the blood, before we're struggling with intractable obesity, and before we have to take a lot of medications.

Unfortunately, prevention is not the focus; the focus lies in "managing" all these metabolic diseases and conditions *downstream* from where insulin resistance started—i.e. after we're in poor metabolic health. Until we address insulin resistance and its dietary cause—too much carbohydrate, especially sugar, starches, flours, etc.— these metabolic diseases are going to continue to skyrocket across the globe. There has been no improvement in diabetes care at the population level in the last 10 years; obesity and hypertension are increasing across all groups. The news keeps getting worse regarding our metabolic health.

High blood sugar resulting from insulin resistance does a lot of damage throughout the body that may not show up until it's really bad—e.g. retinopathy, vascular problems, hearing loss, heart disease, heart attacks, but *these processes are underway in the "prediabetes" range* according to current science.

Thus, in taking control of your carbohydrate consumption, increasing your functional activity and movement, dedicating yourself to getting good sleep each and every night, and taking steps to reduce stress as much as you can, you are *profoundly altering your future*. It sounds dramatic, but insulin resistance is serious; the great news is that when we address it through diet and a few changes in lifestyle, the body responds! It may take some time, but you will see significant improvement.

Remember, it takes a long time for each person to develop insulin resistance followed by prediabetes; but in following the steps in this book, you can reverse it.

Eating Too Much and Too Often

If we continue to eat a diet high in carbohydrate, especially refined carbs/processed foods, sugars both natural and processed, *and* we continue to eat too often as well as too much food because the insulin resistance is making us hungry all the time—a diet that consistently drives up blood sugar—what we're doing is prompting our bodies to pump out more insulin all the time, which drives insulin resistance. As we've discussed this is a vicious cycle.

We break this cycle by limiting consumption of carbohydrate, eliminating sugar in all forms, increasing movement, getting quality sleep, and reducing stress. The biggest factor—*by far*—is controlling intake of carbohydrate, especially sugar and foods that become sugar quickly in the body, which includes "whole grains," all other flours, starchy vegetables, most fruits, and all forms of sugar and artificial sweeteners.

Snacking and eating at all hours is a significant reason we've become insulin resistant as a population. It's not the calories doing this. Eating over long periods by snacking forces our bodies to pump out insulin for extended periods. Studies have shown that since the 1980's in the U.S. we eat a lot more often and consume bigger portions; we snack all the time, a process driven by advertising and even the ADA (American Diabetes Association), which says snacking helps to keep blood sugar "stable." All this snacking increases insulin resistance, which means that it's *destabilizing* your blood sugar over time. All this snacking and larger portions mean our bodies are forced to churn out more insulin day after day.

If we're not following the strict lowest-carb diet, the keto diet, what actually prevents swings in blood sugar is eating a high fiber, low/er carbohydrate, and micronutrient–rich diet with good protein and adequate fat, including saturated fat. Eating natural sources of fat, including saturated fat, helps stabilize blood sugar and insulin levels because it makes us feel full, and it slows the rise in blood sugar. Fat was the treatment for Type 1 diabetes until the invention of exogenous insulin in 1921. If one is *not* on the ketogenetic diet one shouldn't eat enormous amounts of fat because it can blunt the insulin response—but we shouldn't fear saturated from natural sources vis-à-vis heart disease or weight gain.

The problem comes when we eat a diet that's *both* high in carbohydrate *and* fat. It's this combination—high carb *and* high fat together—that's a problem. If we decrease our carbs substantially, most especially refined/processed carbs that really spike blood sugar and insulin such as breads, pastas, cereals, grains, fruit/juice, flours, corn, potatoes, etc., we *can* eat more fat. The key thing to remember is that eating excessive carbs and fat together that causes weight gain—and that's due to the carbs *preventing us from burning fat as a fuel source and releasing fat (weight loss).* Our bodies will burn glucose if it's there, as we've discussed.

The body understands it needs to use what it can't store. Since the body can store fat for later, that's what it does. If our glucose levels in the blood are high from all the carbs and especially sugar, and our bodies are churning out too much insulin in response, the body stores all the excess glucose as fat to be used later as fuel. This means we're not going to burn the fat we consume either; that gets stored too.

The problem is that in the standard American diet "later" never comes for most of us because we're eating far too many carbs all the time, especially processed foods, sugar/fructose—and we're snacking throughout the day and eating into the night when our bodies are designed through evolution to do other important tasks, not deal with food. This constant intake of carbohydrate, especially sugar, for long periods is what *prevents* our bodies from burning fat. This combination of high levels carbs and fat *together* is called an **obesogenic diet**; it makes us fat, diabetic, hypertensive, and it drives cardiovascular disease, NAFLD, and dementia among other conditions and diseases. It is the standard American diet.

Low-fat and calorie-reduction diets are *not* the answer because they don't address the actual problem, which is insulin resistance. Low-carb eating is what addresses the root cause, insulin resistance; as a result, low-carb eating stabilizes blood sugar, blood pressure, cholesterol, and lets us lose weight safely. Metabolically, low-carb is what *allows* our body to release stored fat—i.e. lose weight *without gaining it back.* Our glucose and insulin levels have to be low enough for our bodies to start releasing our stored fat. In other words, you don't have to be on the keto diet for your body to do this; you just have to be eating under *your specific level of carbohydrate tolerance.*

Finding your personal carb tolerance level can take some time, but by measuring your blood sugar regularly throughout the day for a couple of weeks, especially in response to food and exercise, you will get a clear picture of your personal level of carbohydrate tolerance—i.e. what you can eat, what you can't, and how you need to exercise in order to stabilize blood sugar and insulin levels consistently.

The combination of high carbs *and* high fat causes us to store more fat. A low-carb and high fat diet *does not cause us to store fat.* The human body won't release fat from our fat cells, and it won't burn fat from the diet for fuel, unless and until we lower our glucose and insulin levels sufficiently. This is just the way the body works. Bringing down your carbohydrate consumption significantly, especially by eliminating all processed foods and drinks with sugar (natural or artificial), means your body is far better able to release stored fat *and* use the fat you consume for energy. (In other words, one doesn't have to be on the strict keto diet all the time; one can drift in and out of ketosis through a low carb but not necessarily keto diet. In all likelihood, this is how we spent most of our time prior to the invention of agriculture—drifting in and out of ketosis.)

It's also critical for weight loss and restoring insulin sensitivity to eat whole, nutrient-dense, fiber-rich foods that trigger our body's evolutionary responses (i.e. hormonal signals) that tell us we're full.

Processed foods do the opposite: they trigger us to keep eating. You will be surprised at how quickly a diet of whole foods and low sugar/carbohydrate makes you feel so much more full and decreases your cravings! This is simply because our bodies *are designed* to eat this kind of food, not processed foods or loads of sugar (including natural sugars), etc.

Because sweet foods are actually quite rare in nature and contain far less sugar than cultivated fruits we now eat, we're just not adapted from an evolutionary perspective to have a constant supply of sweet foods and drinks. This is the reason we crave sweetness; it's built into us to pay much more attention to sweet foods *because* they're rare in nature. That's how we evolved. Our bodies understand sweet foods as chance to eat a lot of them so we can become *temporarily* insulin resistant—and store all that excess glucose (sugar) as fat. Keep in mind what we discussed earlier; the human species *prioritizes* fat storage as a survival mechanism. Some people store fat better than others from an evolutionary perspective.

Thus, we're wired to pay attention to sweet foods because it's a chance to store fat. This is an ancient, evolutionary impulse in us, and it's one that's very hard to resist. The problem lies in the fact that we now have constant access to sugar and to easily digestible carbs that turn into sugar quickly as well as to artificial sweeteners that make us pump out insulin even though there's no sugar for the insulin to usher into cells.

The body *thinks* there's sugar because of the intense sweetness, so it pumps out insulin. This why artificial sweeteners and various alternative sweeteners contribute to insulin resistance even if they don't raise blood sugar directly. Artificial sweeteners also increase our cravings/addictions for sweet foods/drinks—exacerbating our natural instinct to seek out and overeat sweet food. Millions of years of evolution mean we can't trick our bodies with artificial sweeteners. It just doesn't work.

Some cultures do eat a lot of high-fiber, starchy carbs such as yams and other tubers, but they are also the cultures in which people are (or were) constantly moving and get enough sleep. In other cultures people eat a lot of pasta, but they also have a tradition of walking after meals and throughout the day, which helps to push the glucose from the bloodstream into the muscles where it's used for energy—i.e. movement helps support insulin sensitivity. It's the combination of high sugar/carb diet, lack of sleep, high levels of stress *and* lack of movement that is so deadly.

So, all these snacks and bigger portions, far more processed foods and carbs, high levels of sugar and artificial sweeteners, and the ridiculous (and entirely unscientific) "low fat" nonsense of the 1980's onward have increasingly driven our bodies to pump out insulin all the time. During the early stages of this low-fat craze companies also added a lot more sugar, artificial sweeteners, cheap "vegetable" oils (i.e. light machine oils), and salt to prepared and processed foods in order to compensate for the lack of fat in terms of flavor. These products are the worst things we can eat, and they perpetuate carb and sugar addiction in the human species.

These processed foods tap into our evolutionary vulnerabilities—our inherent desire for sweet foods and foods that turn quickly into sugar such as flours and grains—and as a country we've come to expect more sweetness as well as the immediate availability of cheap, refined food (carbs) in vast quantities.

We expect bigger portions at every meal and "staples" such as potatoes and bread. Potatoes are the most common vegetable eaten by children in this country, and coupled with the above factors, it's no wonder children and adolescents now get "adult onset" diabetes. Potatoes turn into glucose *very quickly*, which spikes blood sugar and insulin in response. From a metabolic standpoint, potatoes should *not* be a staple of our diets. Babies are also getting high levels of sugar in many baby foods and drinks, so this process of spiking insulin and blood sugar now starts in infancy.

The size of the snack industry increased significantly from the 1970's onward and created an entire new meal category (the "snack") comprised mostly of processed and packaged foods filled with refined carbs, sugars, and dangerous "vegetable" oils that are industrial byproducts. (They're machine oils that humans should never consume.) Essentially the snack food industry *is* the obesogenic industry.

Unfortunately, the health food industry that also started in the 1960s and 70's as a reaction to these bad food trends and agricultural abuses now follows this same formula of processed foods and snacks with products that are high in natural sugars such as raisins, dates, and figs. These are better nutritionally than refined sugar or artificial sweeteners and refined grains, but they're still sugar from a metabolic standpoint, and they will still cause insulin resistance and Type 2 diabetes as well as high blood pressure and weight gain.

What's made things far worse is that we no longer have the critical and extended periods of time when our bodies can recover from insulin secretion in response to intake of food and drinks, which is driving insulin resistance across the population—exactly like antibiotic resistance. Our bodies are not designed to metabolize food and drink over many hours of the day. That's not how we evolved as a species, so it's extremely hard on our bodies to do this.

The result is that we have high levels of glucose and insulin circulating in our systems for much longer periods, which is driving metabolic diseases and conditions, including cardiovascular disease and dementia. The brain cannot cope with high levels of sugar—it kills brain cells.

With regard to prediabetes, diet and exercise have consistently been shown to work *better* than Metformin, a first-line drug. Instead of medication, you can control your intake of carbohydrate, use functional exercise, and lower your blood sugar and insulin secretion by not snacking or grazing. The advantage here is that you're actually building insulin sensitivity—i.e. you are actually reversing the disease of (pre)diabetes itself, significantly improving your heart and brain and liver health as well as your immune system.

Insulin injections are a key treatment for Type 2 diabetes; but this exogenous insulin works by *forcing* the sugar out of the blood and *into* the organs and tissues. It force-feeds organs and cells with the high sugar from the bloodstream that comes from diet. Insulin injections also cause weight gain because insulin is the fat storage hormone whether in its natural or synthetic forms. It is important to know that insulin injections as a treatment for diabetes *do not remove* this excess high blood sugar from the body or stop the harm it causes including cardiovascular disease and heart attacks, but insulin makes the A1C test results look better. *The underlying disease of insulin resistance doesn't get better; it gets worse when we force-feed sugar into our organs and cells where it continues to cause damage, including heart attacks.*

This is why Type 2 diabetics need to use more and more medications and insulin—i.e. it gets harder and harder to *force* the sugar from a high carbohydrate diet into the organs and cells where it still causes serious health problems—even as the A1C test looks better. These problems include retinopathy, amputations due to vascular compromise, high blood pressure, heart attacks, strokes, cognitive problems, etc.

Forcing the excess sugar into our organs and cells just makes the underlying insulin resistance much worse. This is why Type 2 diabetes is called a "progressive" disease. It's not a progressive disease—it's a disease that gets worse if we don't address what's causing it, insulin resistance, and if we continue to eat a high carb diet and use insulin to force more and more sugar into cells and organs that are already too full of sugar and resistant to insulin.

Dietary changes such as eating whole foods, limiting carbohydrate intake, *not eating any refined carbs or sugar*, and paying attention to *timing as well as volume of food and balancing macronutrients at every meal* along with exercise, stress reduction, good sleep habits and not snacking are what stop the ever-worsening feedback loop of high blood sugar and insulin resistance. This is *very different* than using medications to force high levels of glucose into cells so the A1C test looks better. That's just hiding the problem so it doesn't show up in the A1C test while making Type 2 diabetes *a lot worse*.

When you eat a diet of whole foods and limit your carbohydrate intake to high fiber natural foods such as above ground vegetables, beans/legumes (if you can tolerate them), nuts and seeds, and pay attention to the amount and timing of food you consume, your cravings and hunger *will* go way down, which is because the body starts to become more insulin sensitive and its hormonal signals of satiety begin working properly again—i.e. high insulin levels no longer block the brain from "seeing" the hormone leptin—which signals satiety. This is the process that breaks the feedback loop of insulin resistance and stops the addictive cravings for refined carbohydrates, especially sugar.

A1C test

The HbA1c test shows the % of sugar bonded to the hemoglobin protein in the blood. This sugar-bonded blood is circulating throughout the body and in all organs and affecting numerous systems and tissues including the vascular system and heart. Hemoglobin cells are replaced every 2-4 months, hence the 3-month window of the A1C test. High blood sugar is literally marinating our organs and cells.

As the body's cells become resistant to the hormone insulin, and fat cells become distended and even more resistant to insulin, the fat cells themselves become estrogenic –i.e. they are not hormonally neutral—and fat cells in the body become yet another factor increasing insulin resistance.

The HbA1c test is an average, and does not show all the daily spikes in blood sugar, which cause damage in the body. It also does not measure insulin resistance, which requires separate testing. (If you're in the prediabetic range, you have insulin resistance. But not all people with insulin resistance have high blood sugar.)

Thus, you should talk to your MD about testing your insulin resistance directly; the more information you have, the better you can understand this underlying root cause of diabetes and prediabetes: insulin resistance. You need to know how bad your insulin resistance is. That will tell you how much you need to control your intake of carbs and how much you will need to exercise to help restore your insulin sensitivity.

High Blood Glucose, High Cholesterol, High Blood Pressure

As we've seen, in the state of insulin resistance cells become less able to take up and use glucose from the blood, which ends up getting stored as fat in several places in the body, primarily the liver, followed by the pancreas, cells, etc., and then it pools in the blood as the last stop on the insulin-resistance train. Weight gain increases, hunger escalates, hormonal signals that tell us we're full don't work properly, blood pressure and triglycerides rise, vessels stiffen, fat cells release more hormones (estrogen) that worsen insulin resistance and so on. This threatens the health of our hearts and brains.

All of this happens because we consume too much dietary carbohydrate, primarily in the form of processed foods, simple sugars, flours and grains, starchy vegetables like potatoes and corn, and we eat far too often. Refined, "enriched" bread does not grow on trees, and we can't dig pasta out of the ground. Anything can be called "whole grain." Our bodies are *not adapted to processed foods* from an evolutionary perspective, and they're not adapted to sedentary lifestyles. Most especially our bodies are not adapted to the lethal combination of high blood sugar/high insulin, lack of movement, lack of sleep, and too much stress.

Finally, our current Dietary Guidelines for Americans actually recommend everyone eat many servings a day of grains and too much fruit and up to 10% of calories in sugar—which anyone with high blood sugar, insulin resistance, or any problems with metabolic health should *not* be doing. The DGA says this because certain nutrients have been added back to refined grains *after being removed in the first place* during the refinement process (!) and because the DGA tells us to limit red meat and saturated fat (based on *very weak* epidemiological evidence), which are excellent sources of precisely these nutrients.

In other words, the DGA tells us to stop eating the animal foods that we've been eating as a species during the millions of years of our evolution when most of our genes were established and instead to eat refined, toxic junk that turns into sugar very quickly and causes insulin resistance over time.

We're *designed* to eat animal foods; this is our evolutionary history as a species. If we choose to be vegetarian or vegan we need to supplement carefully and control our carbs by not eating refined, processed carbs and limiting sugary fruits and starchy vegetables. We also need to eat natural sources of fat such as olive oil, coconut, nuts and seeds, and avocados so we're getting enough saturated fat. We *evolved* eating saturated fat! Since the 1980s the idea has been that saturated fat is terrible for us.

This *hypothesis*, which has never been proven, was based on *very* bad science decades ago. It then became an entrenched *myth* for many reasons that include politics, economics, and personality conflicts within the sciences—in other words robust science is not the basis on which this unproven, pervasive belief is founded. Our entire evolutionary history tells us saturated fat is not the problem. How the human body works tells us this too. The fact that we can use dietary fat as well as glucose for energy tells us this.

We can get all the nutrients we need for good health *without* eating refined grains/ carbohydrates— if we focus on a whole and real food diet—as well as enough fat (including saturated fat) to make many of these vitamins and nutrients bioavailable to us (e.g. vitamins A, E, D, and K, which are **fat soluble** vitamins.) Although it's more challenging to do and requires some careful supplementation, vegetarians and vegans can definitely get all the essential vitamins and nutrients necessary for good health without consuming animal products *or* the refined grains, sugar, and excessive levels carbohydrates that worsen blood sugar and insulin resistance.

If we're not using it for energy, the body has to store all this excess glucose from dietary carbohydrate as fat, which results in high triglycerides. High triglycerides are especially dangerous because they are smaller molecules that get under the lining of the blood vessels, narrowing and stiffening them. The bigger, "fluffy" cholesterol molecules produced in response to food such as eggs and cheese and meat are actually *far* less harmful and dangerous. Most of these are cleared from the body. In other words, they are there but they are not doing damage. It's when cholesterol molecules *get bonded with sugar* that they become a problem.

So, the DGA should be taking actual facts into consideration before recommending that *everyone* eat a diet that's high in carbohydrate and that includes refined, toxic grains and flours, as well as up to 10% of our diet in sugar, toxic "vegetable" oils, far too little natural fat, not enough meat, etc.

Similarly, high blood pressure is also the body's response to excessive dietary carbohydrate as well as high intake of salt for those who are sensitive to it, which is only about 20% of people, lack of appropriate nutrients, lack of exercise, etc. High blood pressure and high blood sugar (glucose) also worsen one another in a process of vascular "remodeling" that strongly influences diabetic complications.

Thus, people with high blood pressure must limit intake of dietary carbohydrate, most especially sugar, refined grains, flours, processed foods, and sugary fruits. Again, any set of national dietary guidelines should not recommend high levels of dietary carbohydrate for everyone given that it's not an essential part of the diet like protein or fat.

Given that only 12% of Americans are metabolically healthy[9], 88% of us should not be eating high levels of carbs, processed foods, refined grains and flours, juice, or starchy vegetables like potatoes—let alone foods with added sugar or sweeteners in any form.

---

[9] Joana Araújo, Jianwen Cai, and June Stevens. Metabolic Syndrome and Related Disorders. Feb 2019. ahead of print http://doi.org/10.1089/met.2018.0105

What High Blood Sugar Feels Like

Supposedly there are no symptoms of prediabetes. This is not true if you pay attention to the underlying cause: insulin resistance. You can feel insulin resistance if you know that what's going on is not "getting older" or "natural decline."

Insulin resistance causes food cravings and frequent hunger, especially for simple carbs (i.e. quick sugar) because our cells aren't getting the glucose they need due to insulin resistance, and insulin resistance is blocking the brain's ability to "see" leptin, the satiety hormone. Insulin resistance causes weight gain and increased eating in an attempt to get glucose into the cells as well as to keep blood sugar from crashing.

Unlike protein or fat, carbohydrate is addictive to most humans, most especially sugar in any form. As we discussed, carbohydrate and sweet foods in particular were not common throughout in our evolutionary experience, so resisting them is difficult for us. We're wired to consume them if we can; the reason for this is because they provide us with an opportunity to spike our blood sugar and store that excess glucose as fat—*temporary* insulin resistance.

From an evolutionary perspective, our interest in sweet foods makes sense. They provide us with a chance to *store fat* for survival. Now that these foods are absolutely are everywhere in our lives, it's extremely difficult for us to ignore them. We no longer have long periods (weeks or months) when we don't consume them, so our bodies are overwhelmed.

Insulin resistance causes that "hangry" feeling due to blood sugar swings. High blood sugar affects memory, cognitive functioning, mood, and concentration. The science is clear that high blood sugar and insulin resistance affect the brain in very significant ways. As you get your blood sugar and insulin response under control, your energy will improve, and mental fog and confusion will lessen. Cognitive focus and short-term memory will also improve.

Addressing high blood sugar and insulin resistance has important ramifications for brain health and cognitive functioning—both now and in the future. High sugar kills brain cells, so it's not surprising that we suffer a range of brain and mood problems if our brain is marinating in sugar.

Summary of Causes of Insulin Resistance

Too much dietary carbohydrate doesn't make you feel full, especially those processed foods that dump sugar into the bloodstream quickly; to the contrary these foods *increase* hunger, blood sugar swings, and cravings. Processed foods have little to no nutritional value, fiber, protein, etc., and they do not trigger the chemical signals in our bodies to stop eating. Processed foods are easily digestible carbohydrates, which cause increased hunger and cravings for more carbohydrates and especially sugars. Unlike refined and processed "food," real and whole foods trigger satiety (hormonal signaling processes) that tells us we're full.

Causes of insulin resistance:

1.) Excessive and chronic stimulation of insulin secretion in the body by eating too often and too much carbohydrate, especially refined grains and flours, sugar in all forms, and fructose—especially in sodas/drinks and processed foods, and artificial/alternative sweeteners that prompt insulin secretion

2.) Excess weight—especially belly fat

3.) Lack of exercise (exercise helps insulin push the glucose into the cells and makes them more sensitive to insulin)

4.) Stress (release of cortisol)

5.) Lack of sleep

Other factors that can affect blood sugar and insulin levels to a lesser degree include:

Toxins in food, environment (e.g. BPA-lined cans linked to diabetes, endocrine-disrupting pesticides on food)

Excessive amounts of dietary fat blunting the effectiveness of insulin in the body, if you're not on the ketogenic diet or eating a low enough carb diet

Genetics

All of these factors operate individually and as a feedback loop; they amplify the effects of one another. By paying attention to #1-5 above, you will significantly improve your blood sugar and reverse the underlying disease, insulin resistance, causing it. You will cure yourself.

Diabetes also doesn't have to be "progressive"—it's a feedback loop, which worsens over time. "Progressive" and feedback loop *are different things*. The former is *inevitable*; the latter can be broken if you break each link in the feedback loop by addressing each cause of insulin resistance and its resultant high blood sugar—beginning with #1-5 above.

The Essential Dietary Steps to Reversing Prediabetes

Step One: The first step is to *eliminate intake of foods and other substances that spike blood sugar and insulin levels*, i.e. stop the intake of excess dietary carbohydrate, including natural sugar. Get rid of the worst offenders first, the ones that do the most damage, and this will make a huge difference.

Get rid of these first:

All ultra-processed foods, *which are just another form of sugar*. If you don't make it, or it's not in mostly in a natural form (e.g. an apple, a chicken breast, a fish fillet, a stalk of broccoli), don't eat it.

All refined sugar, artificial sweeteners, and alternative sweeteners: e.g. white sugar, brown sugar, corn syrup, all artificial sweeteners in any form/any brand, and all alternatives such as agave, etc. Read labels to be sure you're not getting sugar alcohol or other sugar substitutes that spike insulin even if they don't spike blood sugar directly. A lot of "sugar free" foods do this to avoid having to list "added sugar" to nutrition labels, but things like sugar alcohol and artificial sweeteners and sugar "alternatives" that spike insulin response *will* worsening insulin resistance—even if they're technically "sugar free." Remember, "sugar free" is just a marketing gimmick designed for product labels; it does not tell us what happens inside our bodies once we ingest this stuff.

This also means no diet drinks. These trick the body into pumping out insulin, and we do not want to make the body pump out insulin all the time. Through hormonal signaling that begins with what we taste on our tongues, our brains quickly believe we've just eaten something *really* sweet. The body rapidly prepares by releasing insulin to deal with what it believes will be a big spike in blood sugar. Then there's no spike in blood sugar; yet, the body has just pumped out all this insulin.

This false alarm makes the cells ignore insulin (i.e. causes insulin resistance) when they're constantly flooded with insulin for no reason. It makes the cells refuse to answer the door when insulin comes knocking. This worsens insulin resistance, which drives pre/diabetes. Get rid of all artificial sweeteners! (Originally they were invented for Type 1 diabetics, who don't produce insulin. In Type 2 diabetes, including prediabetes, the body does produce insulin.)

All natural sugar in liquid form, such as honey, fruit juice, and molasses. This is because sugar in liquid form has no fiber and enters the blood stream *very* quickly spiking blood sugar and insulin secretion.

White potatoes

White rice and brown rice

Corn

Wheat

These are the primary dietary offenders that cause blood sugar spikes. *Controlling blood sugar over time is all about controlling blood sugar spikes and insulin spikes*. Over the course of 2-4 months, your average blood sugar will come down, and your A1C will improve. Your carbohydrate tolerance will also improve so that the carbs you do consume such as above ground vegetables, berries, tomatoes, and avocados affect your blood sugar less and less. This is what happens as your insulin sensitivity improves—i.e. insulin is far more efficient in moving that glucose from the carbs you do eat into your cells to be used for energy.

The most important thing is the fact that you won't be pumping out insulin all the time in response to food, so your cravings will start to go way down. You'll also stop storing all that excess glucose as fat. Also, you need to avoid artificial sweeteners of any kind as most spike insulin levels—and controlling blood sugar and weight is all about reversing the root cause: insulin resistance.

Making these changes in your diet takes time. This is about improving insulin sensitivity for the rest of your life and therefore preventing diabetes, cardiovascular disease, and brain disorders. It takes some time to make these dietary and lifestyle changes, but they will alter your future in profound ways.

Above all, this is not a crash or fad calorie-counting diet that will only make things worse by permanently slowing your metabolism, making you more interested in food, and less interested in exercise. This is what the body does in response to perceived starvation, which is what every calorie-counting diet is. Remember that calories aren't the problem; insulin resistance is the problem.

In terms of improving your blood sugar and insulin resistance, remember that A1C test is an average; it does not show the daily spikes in blood sugar that do damage or show you your insulin levels. Eliminate simple carbs, grains and flours—including "whole grains," starchy vegetables, and sugar in all forms, your metabolic health, including your blood sugar, will improve very quickly.

Remember that carbohydrate is the only macronutrient (vs. protein and fat) that raises blood sugar significantly. It's also the only entirely *optional* macronutrient. We must eat protein. We must eat fat. We don't have to eat carbs. Our bodies are designed this way through evolutionary processes. You have a choice whether to eat any carbohydrate, how much carbohydrate to eat, and which carbs to eat. You must eat protein, *and you must eat fat*: <u>both</u> are necessary to our bodies.

Start with what you can eliminate most easily in Step One. Then decrease your intake of other items above that might be harder such as wheat (bread, pasta, etc.). Continue to reduce your intake of each until you're not eating anything in Step One.

As you eliminate each thing *replace it with a better substitute such as animal protein (including fish), nuts and seeds, limited dairy/cheese, veggies, beans (if your blood sugar can tolerate them), and fat,* etc. Swap white potatoes for limited baked sweet potatoes, which have a lot of fiber and micronutrients, but don't eat them too often, and don't eat a lot at a time because they are high in natural sugar.

If Step One, eliminating these biggest offenders, takes a few weeks to accomplish, *that's fine*. It's *far better to eliminate these worst offenders permanently* in terms of their disproportionate effect on your blood sugar. Processed foods in particular take less time to eat (i.e. less time to chew and swallow) and less time to digest, so the sugar spikes in your bloodstream much faster—and then the insulin spikes follow.

Ultra-processed foods such as potato chips, crackers, cakes, bread, pasta, candy, etc. *don't* trigger the chemical signals in our bodies that tell us we're full, so our brains don't get the message to stop eating. These substances also don't fill our stomachs in terms of either volume or energy density in the way real food does, which means our brains don't get the signals from the stomach that we have eaten as much as we have. These foods are designed this way so we'll keep eating them.

Thus, we can continue to eat large amounts of ultra-processed foods (especially sugar, refined grains, flours, and starches) without ever feeling full. Ultra-processed foods don't exist in nature, and over millions of years of our evolution we weren't exposed to them, so our stomachs and brains and chemical signaling processes can't deal with them effectively or accurately; further, these processed substances are *designed to trigger the addictive centers in the human brain*, so we will continue to eat more of them. This is the profit motive at work in triggering our evolutionary vulnerabilities like this.

We want to eat these substances because we're wired through evolution to pay more attention to foods that turn quickly into sugar in the body—i.e. at an evolutionary level, we understand these foods provide us with a chance for our bodies to store all this excess glucose as fat. This *isn't* going on at a conscious level; we crave these foods for evolutionary reasons that are millions of years in the making.

Remember, evolution has taught us over millions of years that storing fat is an important priority, which is why we are so driven to eat sweet foods and processed foods that we store so easily as fat. Since the mid-twentieth century, these foods have become far more available in all types of environments, and the culture has changed so much that eating/snacking is now encouraged in all kinds of settings. Finally, because many health and diabetes-related groups are funded by processed food and drug companies, we're getting "advice" based on deep financial and ideological conflicts of interest.

If we don't feel full for a considerable period of time after eating, it's very likely because the we're eating foods that bypass the hormonal signaling processes in our bodies—e.g. Processed foods, grains and flours, sugar in all forms, etc. When we eat real food (veggies, meat, fish, fat, nuts, etc.) that's complex and takes time to digest, these chemical signals kick in to tell us we're full, and we do feel full.

You *will* feel full on meat, fish, fat, limited dairy without sweeteners of any kind, good carbs such as hummus and veggies and lentil soup, nuts/seeds. You will *never* feel full on "whole grains," processed foods, excessive fruits, potatoes, corn, etc. These spike our blood sugar and insulin levels but leave us hungry. If you're not eating enough natural fat, you will get hungry.

A word of warning: as you eliminate the foods in Step One, you may experience what's informally called "the carb flu." It's also called the "keto flu" for those who restrict carbohydrate intake more significantly in order to achieve and maintain nutritional ketosis. To remedy this, use much more salt, and eat more avocadoes, leafy greens, and pumpkin seeds for potassium and magnesium.

If you feel lethargic, dizzy, or you experience muscle cramps, it's due to loss of sodium, which happens when you control intake of carbohydrate. (This loss of sodium is called **natriuresis**.) The reason for the carb or keto "flu" (**natriuresis)** is because once insulin levels come down in response to lower intake of dietary carbohydrate, the kidneys don't store water as they do when our blood sugar and insulin levels are high.

Kidneys store water in response to high insulin levels; they do this to try and protect the body from the harm of high insulin that comes with eating a diet that has toxic levels of carbohydrate. Thus, when we begin normalizing our insulin levels, the kidneys start releasing all this excess water that they no longer need to store. When insulin levels come down in the body, the kidneys no longer need to protect the body by storing all this water, so they begin releasing it. When this happens, we do lose sodium.

Thus, you *will need to salt your food* in order to replace this lost sodium. When you do, the symptoms of lethargy, dizziness, muscle cramps, etc. will stop. These are signs that you need more sodium. If you prefer, you can use bone broth (preferably homemade) with plenty of salt in it. You should also increase your intake of non-starchy vegetables such as leafy greens that are high in vitamins and minerals.

Step Two: Don't eat sucrose or fructose beside very limited whole fruit. Eating berries is fine because they have a lot of fiber and release their sugar slowly. The more fiber in the fruit you eat, the better. Berries, tomatoes, and avocadoes are excellent choices because they're low in sugar. Try to eat organic fruits if you can because these crops are heavily sprayed with pesticides that are hormone disrupters, which is not what we need when we're trying to get the hormonal problem of insulin resistance under control. Eat other high-fiber fruits such as apples and pears in *very limited portions* until you understand how they affect your particular blood sugar levels.

Step Three: As you substantially decrease your intake of carbohydrate, sugar, and all alternative sweeteners, *increase* your intake of fat, including saturated fat, from natural sources such as butter, lard, ghee, fatty cuts of meat, fatty fish, olive oil, avocados, full-fat cream and milk, olives, coconut, nuts and seeds. **Do *not* eat "vegetable" oils** such as soybean, corn, cottonseed, and canola. Do not eat butter substitutes; they're often marketed as having olive oil, but if you read the ingredients, they're full of toxic vegetable oils. *Don't eat a butter substitute*—eat butter! The human body metabolizes butter just fine; it won't clog your arteries—that's a myth. The human body can't metabolize "vegetable" oils properly.

Although they're called "vegetable" or "plant-based" oils, they are light machine oils made through extensive industrial and chemical processes; they are very toxic to the human body. We did not evolve over millions of years eating light machine oils. When we cook with them they produce hundreds of other chemical byproducts that are extremely dangerous to our vascular health in particular. Natural sources of *saturated* fat are *stable* fats; "saturated" just means stable—it has to do with the chemical composition of the type of fat. It does not mean "bad;" *it means stable*. That means the human body recognizes and can metabolize it properly.

Step Four: Balance the 3 macronutrients at every meal: 1.) protein 2.) carbs such as above ground vegetables, 3.) good fat (avocados, olive oil, omega 3 fatty acids in fish and flax seeds, saturated fat from meat and dairy if you consume animal products, etc.) This *complexity and balance* at each meal means the body doesn't get a lot of carbs at once, and the body is busy digesting protein and breaking down fat. This means the body turns carbohydrate into sugar more slowly when eaten with protein and fat and a lot of fiber.

Step Five: Do not overcook vegetables, which makes them release their sugar, and eat fat with vegetables. Eat vegetables raw, or al dente, so your body has to work to break them down—along with some fat such as avocado or olive oil. Make your body do the work of breaking food down, which lowers the blood sugar spike from the carbs you eat, which lowers insulin secretion. Be sure to include some fat from natural sources (not "vegetable" oils, which are light machine oils). We *need* fat in order to absorb important vitamins in veggies and the limited fruit we eat such as berries, tomatoes, and avocadoes. *Fat won't make you fat*!

Step Six: Do not eat overly ripe fruit because sugar increases *significantly* with ripeness. Again, focus on berries, tomatoes, and avocadoes until your insulin sensitivity is restored. After that, fruits other than berries, tomatoes, and avocados should be treated as a dessert—an occasional event.

Step Seven: Pay attention to the order in which you eat foods. If you can, eat protein first, which is digested in the stomach. Wait 15 minutes to eat carbs (e.g. veggies). This helps reduce the blood sugar spikes. **Never eat carbs alone, even good carbs**. Always have some protein or good fat with them, even when you eat vegetables. A food such as hummus with olive oil is great because the beans are carb, but they're also a protein with a lot of fiber, and the fat from the olive oil also slows down how quickly the beans breakdown into sugar in your bloodstream. An apple with cheese or peanut butter is also a good option—i.e. pair the carb (apple) with protein and fat—*if you can tolerate the carbohydrate in an apple* and beans. You may need to restrict these for a while until your insulin sensitivity is restored.

Again, use your blood sugar meter consistently to see what the blood sugar spike is—that will tell you whether or not something is above your carbohydrate tolerance. One of the reasons to take your sugar regularly is so that you can see that each day is different because of exercise, sleep, etc.; you want to see *the pattern over time* as you make improvements in each area: diet; exercise; sleep; stress reduction.

Step Eight: *Increase your intake of fiber* from sources, which include vegetables, beans, nuts, low sugar fruit such as berries, chia seeds, flax seeds, etc. Fiber, both soluble and insoluble, is a carbohydrate, but it also acts as a speed bump that slows the rise in blood sugar. Fiber also does all kinds of other amazing things in the body and is critical for gut health; fiber is the food source for the gut biome, the "2nd brain" of the body. In the U.S. we eat very little fiber, and increasing your intake from whole food sources will slow blood sugar spikes from food and help your body in all kinds of other wonderful ways.

Dietary fiber (not from supplements) should be 25-30 grams per day from food if you're a woman, 38 grams if you're a man. Two tablespoons of chia seed provide 36% of your daily fiber! Beans provide anywhere from 15-19 grams per cup, so chia and beans should be at the very top of your list daily. Greens such as spinach and kale are excellent sources of dietary fiber as are peas, cauliflower, nuts, apples, pears, blueberries, strawberries, Brussels sprouts, cabbage, avocados, and artichokes. Some people are sensitive to too much fiber, so be sure to respect your body if too much fiber upsets your digestive system and focus on vegetables for fiber rather than beans/legumes.

Step Nine: Do not char or grill meats as the browning process/caramelizing increases the sugar that goes directly into your bloodstream.

Step Ten: You don't have to eat the minute you get out of bed, but fasting until dinner is not a good idea. Some people prefer to eat two meals a day filled with protein and fat and good carbs, so you could eat a hearty meal of protein, fat, and complex carbs once in the late morning and again around dinner, limiting your eating window. A snack in between (protein and fat but no carbohydrate) is acceptable as long as you're not spiking your blood sugar (and therefore your insulin level), and you're not eating across most of the day and night (i.e. long eating window.)

Remember, your body relies on protein and fat to fuel all of its critical functions; carbs are only for energy. If you do eat breakfast, what you eat matters enormously. Do not eat a carbs for breakfast in the morning if you can help it, even complex carbs such as oatmeal. This will spike your blood sugar and insulin levels for the rest of the day. It's best to eat protein and fat in the morning.

Our bodies are *very sensitive* to carbs in the morning, so eat primarily protein such as eggs, fish, chicken, or yogurt (non-sweetened) with chia seeds, nuts, and berries if you want a small amount of carbohydrate. Eating breakfast will stop your liver from raising your blood sugar, which it does to keep the body from becoming hypoglycemic, and if you don't eat carbs in the morning, you're not chasing your blood sugar down all day.

Exercise

Step One: Increase *functional* exercise/movement. This could mean doing things such as parking farther away from a store and walking. Carry your shopping out to your car rather than using a cart. Take the stairs whenever possible. Take 10 minutes to walk around a parking lot before you go into a store and 10 minutes after you finish your errands to walk around it again. Add 10 minutes of walking to other tasks whenever you can during the day until to it adds up to at least 30 minutes.

You can do 3 or 4 ten-minute increments per day, which will have a significant effect over time. As soon as you're able to do so, extend the 10-minute walks to 15 minutes, 20 minutes, and finally to 30 minutes in a single session. *If you can, walk after each meal to blunt the rise in sugar, especially after dinner.*

Make sure you get up every hour to move; sitting all day is very harmful. Even if we workout and go to a gym, sitting undoes a lot of the good we're doing through exercise.

Step Two: Once you have increased your functional exercise by increasing walking or other movement opportunities throughout your day, begin moderate versions of resistance training and HIIT (High-Intensity Interval Training) for brief periods. Resistance training, or strength training, causes the muscles to contract against external resistance. Examples include weight lifting, squats, push-ups, etc., exercises that make your muscles grow stronger. Strength training helps increase our resting metabolism and helps increase insulin sensitivity as well as bone density.

Resistance or strength training helps insulin push the blood glucose into the large muscle groups, so it's particularly good. Focus on strength training that works these large muscle groups such as back, abs, quads, etc. These large muscles need more glucose from your bloodstream, and they don't take it up as quickly as we age. You can use weights or resistance bands or your own body weight in exercises such as pushups and squats. It's especially important to preserve muscle in middle and older age to help increase insulin sensitivity.

HIIT (High-Intensity Interval Training) allows you to burn fat, especially stomach fat, but not lose muscle, increase your metabolism, and improve your cardio health. Even 10 minutes has cardiac benefits when you do HIIT, *which is alternating periods of short, intense exercise with less intense recovery periods.*

Again, you can do 10 minutes per day of HIIT and 10 minutes per day of resistance training and see significant results in terms of blood sugar quickly. 20 minutes of either will give you significant cardiac benefits. HIIT is really a method of challenging the body to do something faster and more intensively such as walking, swimming, or resistance exercises.

Doing exercise after meals blunts the rise in blood sugar and therefore insulin secretion; thus, if you can, do your resistance or cardio exercise after you eat for a double benefit!

There are many excellent resources on both resistance training and HIIT for every fitness level, and when you're doing well in step one above with walking, begin to research resistance and HIIT options that work best for you.

Step Three: increase exercise to 30 minutes daily after you have mastered steps one and two, including HIIT and resistance training. This could take several weeks or even months before you're able to increase to this level, but along the way you will get significant benefits from steps one and two in terms of stabilizing your blood sugar and building insulin sensitivity. It's not about becoming a world-class athlete or "burning" calories; it's about pushing glucose out of the bloodstream into the muscles, improving insulin sensitivity, and benefiting your heart, bones, and immune system—among many other things.

Appropriate Sleep

It is critical that we get enough sleep. We must be especially disciplined about our sleep hygiene. Even one night of less than 5 hours affects us at the cellular level, including our immunity, and regularly getting 5 hours or less of sleep is associated with the highest levels of BMI and weight gain.

Do not skimp on sleep, which is critical for repairing your body's insulin resistance, memory processing and storage during REM sleep, and helping to clear debris from the brain. Do whatever you can to make sleep a top priority. Avoid using devices such as cell phones, tablets, and other electronic devices before going to bed. If you can, develop the habit of putting away these devices *an hour before going to bed.*

Sleep deprivation, which means less than 7 hours per night on a regular basis, is a serious public health problem. For example, about 30% of Americans do not get enough sleep each night, and as many 70 million Americans have chronic sleep problems. Studies show that sleep deficiency increases the risk of multiple diseases including diabetes, obesity, decreased insulin sensitivity, depression, and cardiovascular disease.

The T.H. Chan School of Public Health at Harvard University has a very good overview article on how sleep affects the brain and multiple areas of health, which I encourage you to read. You can find it here:

https://www.hsph.harvard.edu/nutritionsource/sleep/

Reduce Stress

It is also critical that you reduce stress in ways that are *effective for you*. For some people, this can mean practicing mediation; for other people reading a book is relaxing. For many of us, spending time with a pet brings down stress levels considerably. When we reduce stress, we lower the level of cortisol in our system, which is very important. Cortisol is steroid hormone secreted from the adrenal gland. It's behind the "fight or flight" response when we're in danger.

Cortisol makes fat and muscle cells more insulin resistant, and it increases the production of glucose by the liver, i.e. increases blood sugar levels. Chronic stress means cortisol levels become elevated, which worsens both insulin resistance and blood sugar levels. Thus, stress reduction is very important because of its hormonal effects on the body—especially in relation to both blood sugar and insulin levels.

In addition to your preferred methods of stress reduction, spend at least 90 minutes per week outside. Evidence increasingly shows that being outdoors reduces stress, balances hormones, lowers both blood sugar and blood pressure, and improves immunity. Nature improves our bodies on the *cellular level* and does so quickly.

It's critical that you find time to spend outside. <u>Do not use your phone</u>! *The whole point is to let nature absorb your focus and attention*, which is how nature heals us. Ideally you can combine exercise and outdoors time for a double benefit to your blood sugar and insulin sensitivity.

Lose 7-10% of Body Weight

Data show that 7-10% decrease in body weight is the key threshold at which the body begins to show improvement in blood sugar (i.e. starting the good feedback loop in which insulin is better able to get glucose into the cells). It's very important to lose weight at a steady but not extreme pace. Yo-yo diets have dangerous cardiac implications.

As we've discussed, the body tries to default to its highest weight as a survival method. This means it's challenging to lose weight. Don't try to lose more than 1-2 lbs. per week. If you follow the diet and exercise steps in this guide, you will lose weight slowly and have the best chance of keeping it off without causing biological backlash. As we've discussed, counting calories can cause you to focus on low-calorie, high carbohydrate foods that spike blood sugar and insulin levels, foods that turn *into* sugar quickly in the body—sugar that gets stored as fat.

You can try to starve the body through calorie-restriction diets, but doing so will slow your metabolism, make you much less inclined to exercise, and cause you to focus more on food. These are the *evolutionary* responses to calorie restriction, which the human body *perceives* at the metabolic level as famine. Once we stop counting calories, we gain the weight back—and more because we've damaged our metabolism.

Instead, as you significantly decrease your consumption of carbohydrate, make sure you're eating enough fat from natural sources, not "vegetable" oils, and that you're getting enough protein. Remember *both* protein and fat are *essential*: carbohydrate is not. Once you're no longer storing all the excess glucose from a high carb/high sugar diet and your insulin levels come down, your body will start *releasing* its stored fat—i.e. weight loss—*without* slowing your metabolism. This means you will keep the weight off.

Summary

Dietary

Eat only foods that the body must work to digest and metabolize and eliminate all processed foods (the big offenders) and sugar and all artificial sweeteners. Avoid processed meats because they have chemicals and sugar. If you eat meat, choose some fatty cuts to help balance the protein and fat and to increase satiety.

Eat full-fat cheese, yogurt, milk, etc. rather than low- or nonfat dairy, and make sure yogurt isn't sweetened with anything, including fruit.

Don't drink juice, no matter how "healthy" because it lacks its natural fiber and spikes blood sugar and insulin levels quickly. Eat the whole fruit and veggies instead. Stick to fruits such as berries, tomatoes, lemons/limes, and avocados that don't spike blood sugar and insulin. You get vitamins from vegetables, including vitamin C, and we don't need huge amounts of vitamin C—that's a myth. Lemons/limes provide plenty of vitamin C without all the sugar.

Eliminate all wheat, rice, corn, and potatoes—and all the products that contain them. We also don't need all these so-called "whole grains." All grains and flours become sugar in the body, and the more processed they are, the worse they are for both blood sugar and insulin levels. Instead eat small portions of quinoa, oats, beans, and legumes if your blood sugar can tolerate them.

You may have to focus your meals on meat, fish, above ground vegetables and natural fat until your blood sugar and insulin sensitivity are much better; then you can beans, quinoa, etc. back in small portions that don't cause spikes in sugar and insulin levels. Once you rebuild your insulin sensitivity through diet, exercise, sleep and stress reduction, you may be better able to tolerate whole, fiber-filled carbohydrate such as beans, oats, and quinoa in modest portions.

If giving up bread/wheat is particularly difficult, try Ezekiel bread or Dave's bread (in the red package, which has the lowest sugar content) to help you transition off bread. Both are more expensive, but you will be eating as little bread as possible as a transitional step to eliminating bread. Both brands are higher in fiber and other nutrients than most conventional bread.

Remember "whole grains" is a marketing gimmick that has no consistent definition or standard, and it's not a scientific term. Companies can and do call pretty much anything "whole grain" in order to get people to buy products that are definitely not whole grain in any sense. Ezekiel bread is organic, which is important because of the pesticides used on wheat.

Do not overcook veggies as doing so promotes release of sugar that enters more quickly into the bloodstream. Al dente veggies take longer to digest, and the body has to work to break them down. Always eat natural fat with veggies.

Increase fiber intake. Although it's a carbohydrate, fiber acts as a speed bump for blood sugar spikes. You need both soluble and insoluble fiber. The latter can't be digested so it passes through the body and bulks up the stool. Some people are sensitive to fiber for this reason, so be sure to pay attention to how your body responds to a higher fiber diet. Peas are high in both soluble and insoluble fiber. They're starchy—high on the glycemic index—but because of the fiber, they metabolize in the body without spiking blood sugar too much. So, the glycemic index is a good guide, but there are exceptions such as peas because of the fiber.

Focus on consuming vegetables that grow above ground because they are lower in sugar, veggies such as cauliflower, cabbage, broccoli, squash, zucchini, eggplant, mushrooms, Brussels sprouts, green beans, kale and other leafy greens such as spinach. Cook veggies with butter or olive oil so that you absorb the vitamins in them better, which is what fat enables us to do. Add garlic, herbs, etc. and they're all delicious!

Fiber is a key food for bacteria in the gut (2nd "brain"). Microbiome health is critical to hormonal balance, including insulin regulation in the body, which in turn is critical to losing weight and improving insulin over time, lowering blood sugar, etc.; so, eating lots of fiber-filled veggies is great.

Switch to fruit with more fiber such as berries, apples, pears, and avocados. Berries release their sugar slowly because of the fiber in them, and they have important micronutrients, the same ones that give them their color, which have been proven to help with blood sugar regulation. Eat wild or organic berries if possible as berries are typically sprayed with a lot of pesticides. Buy organic apples and pears for the same reason. Mangoes tend to be cleaner. Lemons and limes won't raise your blood sugar like oranges or bananas will.

Again, depending on your starting point in terms of blood sugar and insulin resistance, you may need to eat just berries, avocadoes, lemons/limes, and tomatoes for several months while you rebuild your insulin sensitivity. You should not be eating bananas or other fruits with high levels of sugar. Use your meter consistently, which will tell you if foods are above your carbohydrate tolerance.

Timing of food consumption, combination of foods, and the sequence in which you eat macronutrients are as important as what you eat. Do not eat carbs such as oatmeal alone—if you can tolerate oatmeal. Many people can't tolerate oatmeal until their insulin sensitivity has been restored. Other foods that are high in carbs (e.g. beans) are easier on your blood sugar because they also have protein and fiber. But add fat such as olive oil because beans don't have fat and *you need all 3 macronutrients together at every meal or snack.*

Figuring out how foods such as beans and oatmeal and quinoa affect your blood sugar takes some time, but by testing your sugar regularly you will get a very clear picture of what you can and cannot tolerate vis-à-vis your specific level of carbohydrate tolerance.

Don't eat carbs in the morning—carbs will spike blood sugar in the morning—making blood glucose higher all day and increasing your cravings, etc. Eat protein such as eggs, fish, meats/chicken, etc. Except for the eggs, these are not typical breakfast foods, but eating them in the morning will make a huge difference in controlling your blood sugar and therefore your insulin secretion throughout the day.

Once your blood sugar has stabilized your insulin sensitivity has improved, you might be able to eat small portions of oatmeal, quinoa, beans, etc. again—along with protein and fat—i.e. once your system is doing better processing carbohydrate without spiking blood sugar. But *it takes time* for your body to be able to properly process carbs again such as oatmeal, quinoa, and beans. For many people, oatmeal, quinoa and beans exceed their personal level of carbohydrate tolerance until their insulin sensitivity has been restored, so you need to track your response to these carbohydrates carefully.

Balance protein, fat, carbs at every meal/snack. If you have to do a macronutrient alone—make it protein or protein/fat such as cheese, slice of baked chicken with avocado, etc. Fat helps one feel full, and there's evidence full fat is beneficial, and that those who have a higher level of fat in the diet lose more weight. (What we *cannot* do is combine high intake of fat *with* high intake of carbohydrate; when we do *both*, we gain weight. Eating fat without the carbohydrate is very, very different than eating fat and carbs together.)

Dairy: Evidence indicates that the calcium in dairy helps regulate blood sugar and helps decrease insulin resistance. Be careful not to eat too much, especially yogurt and milk, because of the high level of natural sugar in them. Not all dairy products are the same in terms of effects on blood sugar and insulin. Make sure you do not consume yogurt with any sweeteners—either natural or artificial, and **full fat** is far better than low fat.

Buy organic beans, dairy, meats, fruit and veggies if possible. Wheat, corn, beans, rice, and oats are all sprayed with horrific pesticides in the fields *after* harvest because it's a desiccant and dries these agribusiness crops for processing. Studies show that when pesticides are applied at this last point in the agricultural cycle, *humans ingest a lot more of them*. So, because it's applied after the plant has stopped growing, we're *eating the pesticides directly*. Since you're going to be eliminating processed/prepared foods and drinks, sugar in all forms, and juices as well as wheat, corn, potatoes, and rice, you can use the money you save to make organic choices when possible.

Organic foods lessen the toxic load on the body with fewer hormonal disruptors such as pesticides that increase insulin resistance in the long term. Further, organic meats can't be fed nonorganic grain—e.g. genetically modified corn that's also been soaked in pesticides to dry it out.

Organic foods have higher vitamin and mineral profiles due to being grown in much better soil that hasn't been destroyed by decades of pesticides. Conventional crops are grown in far worse soil, and consequently many conventional crops lack nutrients because these nutrients are not in the soil in which they're grown. A key aspect of food cravings is that processed and nutrient-weak foods grown in poor soil don't satisfy the body at the cellular level. Therefore, one craves other foods in an attempt to get necessary micronutrients, etc.

Again, focus on organic veggies and meats and dairy to the degree possible for your. You will save a lot of money when you're no longer buying expensive and toxic processed foods and drinks, prepared foods, or any of the foods that disproportionately cause metabolic problems over time: sugar; wheat; rice; corn; and potatoes. We eat huge amounts of these as a culture, so replacing these with above ground vegetables, meat/fish, full-fat dairy, natural fat, nuts and seeds will change everything in terms of your blood sugar and insulin levels—and weight loss will take care of itself on this whole food, low sugar, low carbohydrate way of eating. You will also feel a lot less hungry! Remember, carbs make us hungry; protein and fat do not.

Micronutrients

The body "craves" micronutrients, but these cravings trigger a generic response (hunger) that's not very specific. As humans we have one general sensation of "being hungry" either for calories or for specific nutrients. *It's very difficult for a person to tell the difference.* Advertising and marketing make us think that "hunger" is always a matter of wanting more food, and that quick processed foods in huge quantities are the answer. These foods quickly spike blood sugar and insulin levels and combine addictive substances (bad "vegetable" oils, sugar, chemicals, etc.) to keep people eating them. They worsen insulin resistance significantly and increase cravings for more of these foods simply because it's very difficult from an evolutionary perspective for us to resist them.

Because humans can't easily distinguish between hunger and micronutrient insufficiency, often we don't understand that our bodies are craving specific micronutrients. So, when we eat a wide range of low-carb veggies (green, red, purple, orange, white, etc.), protein, fat, and fiber in the form of beans/legumes and quinoa (to the degree we can tolerate these), nuts and seeds, veggies, etc., we increase our intake of important micronutrients that reduce inflammation, relax blood vessels, and provide our cells with the complex nutrients they need. This makes us feel much more satisfied and therefore less hungry. Hunger isn't always about calories; it's very much about nutrients.

Thus, the nutrient density of foods is very important in reducing the craving for foods that are high in carbohydrate (especially sugar) but that are low in the micronutrients we actually need. When we improve our cellular health we feel much less hungry and the cravings go down—most especially when we consume them in low-carb foods that don't send us on a blood sugar rollercoaster. With fish, meat, nuts, enough healthy fat, and a range of non-starchy veggies, very limited fruit, the cravings/hunger will decrease rapidly because our cells are getting what they need *and* we're not subjecting our bodies to a rollercoaster of blood sugar and insulin spikes.

We get hungry quickly if we're not eating enough natural fat such as butter, meat, fish, olive oil, avocados, cheese, etc. (not "vegetable" oils); as we've discussed, fat is *essential* to all humans, so don't skimp on the healthy fat such as olive oil and olives, cheese, fatty meat and fish, and nuts and seeds in limited portions because of the high omega 6 levels—we don't want excessively high levels of omega 6 fatty acids from nuts and seeds in the diet. What we can *never* do is eat a high level of fat *and* a high level of carbohydrate. That's the obesogenic diet, which is the standard American diet.

Focus on Diet for Bioavailable Vitamins and Minerals

Rather than spending money on vitamin and mineral supplements focus on your diet and building food choices and meals around the 10 essential dietary steps and the list of staples in this book, which are the foundation of your weekly food prep and planning. When you're eating enough fat from natural sources, your body will be far better able to absorb important vitamins, many of which are fat soluble.

In specific situations supplementation is necessary. Vegans must use careful supplementation in order to get all the nutrients we need as humans, especially the B complex vitamins. If you have an extremely low level of vitamin D, which is actually a hormone, a deficiency that is *very common* and easily diagnosed with a simple blood test, that deficiency can be remedied quickly, inexpensively, and safely with a vitamin D3 supplement. Ask your MD to order the test.

Remember that you need dietary fat in order for the body to properly absorb some vitamins. Remember, from an evolutionary perspective our bodies are designed to consume a high level of natural fat and an extremely low level of carbohydrate; this means that our bodies need fat in order to make certain vitamins bioavailable—and vitamin D is one of them.

During the pandemic it's especially important to make sure we have enough vitamin D; low levels of this hormone are associated with worse outcomes in response to the disease caused by this virus. If you have adequate levels of vitamin D in your system, overloading on vitamin D won't make a difference in terms of outcomes. In other words, people with significant vitamin D deficiency are at higher risk of complications from the disease caused by this virus.

I do not recommend that you take a multivitamin or other vitamins or minerals unless there's evidence you need them due to deficiency, such as vitamin D, or because you don't eat certain foods such as meat or fish or dairy. Second, our bodies absorb vitamins and minerals from dietary sources far better than from supplements. The reason for this is that dietary sources are far more bioavailable to the human body. For millions of years we didn't take supplements; our bodies evolved to absorb vitamins and minerals from food sources, not pills.

Excessive levels of vitamins and minerals are simply excreted or stored in organs/tissues in ways that can be very *harmful*; for example, for many years women were told to take calcium supplements to prevent osteoporosis. This was bad medical and nutritional advice. Calcium builds up in the soft tissues of the body, including the heart valves, which causes very serious heart problems. If you're eating fish, including the bones in fish such as sardines, consuming cheese and full fat yogurt and milk, etc., and doing *weight-bearing exercise* such as walking, you'll get all the calcium you need, and your body can store it properly in your bones.

If you have far more calcium than your body can store properly because you're taking supplements, it's going to get stored in places such as the heart valves where it should not be stored. When it comes to vitamins and minerals more is not necessarily better, and it can be dangerous. Food is the way we evolved to get necessary vitamins and minerals *in the amounts* we can use and store properly.

When our diet is deficient, such as the vegan diet, then we do need to supplement carefully to make up for what we're not getting through animal products such as many of the B vitamins. Many of us don't get enough vitamin D because we spend most of our time indoors; this wasn't the case during our evolutionary history. Fortunately, we can remedy that common deficiency with a safe supplement that has been studied extensively. Many other vitamins and minerals have not been studied, so it's important not to trust whatever the manufacturers say; they're trying to sell you stuff that you don't need and that could harm you, especially in high amounts.

For example, turmeric is very fashionable at the moment. Used widely in South Asian and other cuisines, *it's meant to be cooked.* These cuisines are thousands of years old, and that's how people have consumed turmeric. Humans barely absorb raw turmeric and its medicinal polyphenol curcumin, and what little we do absorb, we excrete quickly. It can build to toxic levels in the liver if we consume raw turmeric in pill form; it's a very bad idea. Incorporating turmeric *into food and cooking* it is a great idea because *that's how our bodies can absorb and can use it—i.e. along with other foods that increase absorption of curcumin*—and at levels that aren't toxic.

That's how we're meant to eat turmeric—cooked in food via cuisines that have developed over thousands of years—and that's how these cultures use it. One of the spices used in these cuisines regularly is black pepper, which contains piperine that increases the bioavailability of curcumin *significantly—nearly 2000%*. Thus, the best thing you can do is learn to make a few dishes from these cuisines, particularly Indian, and enjoy the benefits of your turmeric the way we are meant to—cooked in food.

Finally, supplements aren't regulated. One can't be sure what is in many of them. Studies have shown a wide range of problems with supplements, which vary from the benign to the very serious, so choose carefully and wisely.

Unless we need to take supplements for specific reasons (e.g. we're vegan, or we're already deficient in a specific vitamin or mineral), we get the best value for our money when we buy excellent, preferably organic, foods (including herbs and spices) and when we dedicate our time and money to preparing diverse meals that are rich in nutrients, including micronutrients. This complexity is what makes us feel full and helps repair the hormonal message system in our bodies, and enables us to properly absorb the vitamins and minerals our bodies need.

The right foods provide a synergistic complexity and bioavailability of vitamins and minerals that supplements can't approximate. The right foods eaten in the right combinations give us the fiber and nutrients our bodies need. Finally, in conjunction with an excellent diet, use appropriate, functional exercise to help reduce inflammation, improve cognition, lower blood sugar, increase insulin sensitivity, and help address high blood pressure and high triglycerides.

Exercise Program

Begin exercise program of moderate exercise 6 days per week for 4-6 weeks, and be very consistent. This is *functional* exercise targeted at getting blood sugar down and increasing your insulin sensitivity—not necessarily "working out" in the athletic sense. If you can and want to work out for longer periods and more intensely that's wonderful. If you're not used to exercising, use functional exercise on a daily basis to push your blood sugar down and to get your cells to become more responsive to the hormone insulin—build insulin sensitivity.

Remember, insulin has more than one job in the body: it facilitates getting glucose into the cells to be used as energy *and* it facilitates fat storage. It can only do one of these two things at a time. When we're insulin resistant glucose doesn't get into the cells properly, *and* insulin prompts our bodies to store all the excess glucose from a high carb diet as fat.

Rebuilding your insulin sensitivity means getting your cells to become more responsive when insulin comes knocking on the (cell) doors, so your cells will answer the door and let the glucose in. However, if you're still eating a high carbohydrate diet, you will continue to overwhelm your cells with glucose.

So, exercise helps your cells answer the door when insulin knocks, and if you're *also* eating a low-carb diet, your cells respond better because they're not already stuffed full of glucose. Thus, exercise helps insulin get the glucose from the bloodstream into the cells rather than prompting the body to store all that glucose as fat. The more you can exercise your large muscle groups such as legs and back the better. The reason for this is that large muscle groups use more glucose from the blood.

In particular, targeted, functional exercise **after meals** will help lower blood sugar spikes after eating and help your insulin move the glucose from your blood into your cells. For example, a very brisk 20 minutes of exercise can drop your blood sugar significantly after dinner, which means that you spend a huge chunk of time better blood sugar and lower insulin, i.e. when you're sleeping. Second, through exercise you're also training your cells to know when insulin is knocking on the door—i.e. you're making your cells more insulin sensitive again.

Functional exercise in the first few weeks will also help build your insulin sensitivity even more as you decrease your intake of dietary carbohydrate, most especially in the form of processed foods and grains and flours, all of which the body turns into sugar, as well as foods with added sugar, juice, sugary fruits, starchy vegetables, and all artificial/alternative sweeteners. Functional exercise will begin to improve your cardiovascular health by addressing the underlying metabolic issues—i.e. insulin resistance and high blood sugar that stiffen blood vessels, drive high blood pressure, etc.

Address the metabolic problems first through dietary strategies and functional exercise. Increase your exercise gradually if you're not used to it; the reason for this is that sudden hard workouts can spike blood sugar, which is not what you want to do.

The point is to get your body to take up glucose more quickly and rebuild insulin sensitivity; it's not about running a 20-mile marathon or swimming the English Channel. Moderate exercise 20-30 minutes after eating is especially beneficial because it gives you longer windows of time when your blood sugar is lower—and because it blunts postprandial blood sugar and insulin secretion.

All exercise helps the body improve insulin sensitivity, and the more consistent you can be the better. If walking is what you can do most easily, do that. If it's too cold or hot to go outside, walk up and down stairs for 15-20 minutes, which gets the large muscle groups in the legs, core, and back to suck up glucose from the bloodstream. Remember, the purpose of this functional exercise is to blunt the rise in blood sugar after meals whenever possible and most of all—to *teach your cells to be insulin sensitive again*—i.e. to listen when insulin comes knocking on the cellular doors trying to usher in glucose from your blood.

The more exercise you can do, the better, but begin where you are and work up to more exercise gradually. *All forms of exercise* will help lower your blood sugar and insulin levels over time, the byproduct of which is weight loss. "Burning" calories is entirely beside the point. As you continue to exercise, you will start to increase your metabolism, which can also increase appetite. As long as you're following the dietary advice in this book, you can include more protein and fat as well as additional above ground vegetables eaten with fat. Amount of food matters, but *blood sugar and insulin spikes matter far, far more* when it comes to controlling weight.

Weight Loss is the Byproduct of Addressing Insulin Resistance

If you're consume a diet low in carbohydrate and exercise so your cells become insulin sensitive again, you will lose weight. This will happen naturally. Exercise alone *cannot* compensate for a diet high in carbohydrate, especially easily digestible carbs (grains and flours) and sugar, and exercise is *not* the primary reason for weight loss, which is an appropriate diet that doesn't prompt your body to store fat through high levels of insulin secretion as well as insulin resistance. Exercise does play a crucial role in building insulin sensitivity, regulating gene expression related to obesity, building cardiovascular health, and making us feel a lot better!

Increasing movement is key in the first few weeks. You also need to give your body a chance to begin healing before making demands on it to work out if you're not used to doing so. Sudden hard workouts can drive blood sugar up and worsen insulin resistance because hard workouts trigger hormonal responses that your blood sugar is taking a sudden nosedive, so the liver "thinks" your body is in crisis and dumps sugar into the bloodstream to "save" you—hence the sudden spike in blood sugar.

This is the flight or fight response at the hormonal level induced by hard exercise when the body is not metabolically ready for hard workouts. Moderate and slowly increasing HIIT will prepare your body for more demanding exercise without triggering this response by the liver and worsening your blood sugar levels.

It's **not possible** to lose much weight through exercise alone via the calories in/calories out model. Do not focus on counting calories, most especially because the body does not use or burn calories. We can talk about calories all we want; the body has no receptors for them. The body understands protein, fat, and carbohydrate—and when we eat—in terms of how it stores fat.

Intermittent fasting does not slow metabolism in the way ongoing calorie restriction does. If you want to try intermittent fasting there are many resources for doing so written by experts, particularly the work of Dr. Jason Fung. You can also get the benefits of fasting by not eating after dinner and not snacking. Both of these things are forms of fasting, and they help stabilize blood sugar and insulin levels.

Eat whole foods, which trigger your hormones that tell you that you're full. Processed food doesn't trigger the hormones that tell our brains we're full: real food does. Don't eat more food once you sense that you're full, and consuming enough fat helps us feel full, but remember not to eat "vegetable" oils like soybean and corn oil: olive, avocado, and coconut oils are fine. Respect that signaling process in your body that has been damaged. It will return with a diet of low-carb, whole foods that align with how we evolved as a species.

Moderate, functional exercise in the first few weeks, especially after meals, blunts blood sugar spikes and therefore stabilizes blood sugar and insulin secretion over time. Increasing your functional exercise consistently *accelerates* this process of restoring your insulin sensitivity. While you're eating foods that don't spike your blood sugar—i.e. your body isn't being overwhelmed with dietary carbohydrate and you're not eating too often—your insulin levels have a chance to come down for long periods.

This dual process results in *inevitable* weight loss because your cells are using more glucose, and you're eating a much lower level of carbohydrate; taken together, your body is being prompted to use glucose rather than store it as fat.

Reducing blood sugar consistently is the most important thing you can do to get the body to stop storing fat. This drives the weight loss. **Well-controlled blood sugar = less insulin secretion = less fat storage = weight loss without evolutionary backlash** (e.g. without slowing metabolism, or making you more interested in food and less interested in exercise, etc.)

Do not sit for more than an hour at a time. Get up and walk for 5-10 minutes and do something that gets your heart rate up a little such as walking up a set of stairs, etc. The cumulative effect of such "exercise snacks" is to repeatedly and consistently blunt the rise in blood sugar and insulin secretion. 20 minutes of brisk walking after lunch and dinner will not cure insulin resistance instantly, but done consistently every day it will lower blood sugar after meals, which in turn means the body releases less insulin. This process builds insulin sensitivity, which means glucose gets into the cells rather than being stored as fat and piling up as high blood sugar.

Remember, exercise helps insulin do its job—i.e. exercise pushes glucose into the cells, especially into the large muscle groups with strength training and HIIT, and long-term, consistent exercise improves insulin sensitivity by making cells far more receptive to insulin again. It helps the "lock" and "key" fit together again—that is, insulin and insulin receptors on the cells—and helps break the feedback loop of insulin resistance.

As you exercise consistently, you will lose weight because insulin is working better—not because you're "burning" calories—and consequently appetite evens out because insulin is getting the glucose into your cells more efficiently to be used for energy. Fat cells in particular become less distended and more receptive to insulin.

Again, don't underestimate the value of "exercise snacks" such as taking stairs, walking 10-20 minutes at lunch at a good pace, take 15-minutes to walk up and down the stairs, etc. It all helps, and you don't need to do "intense" workouts.

Remember, "burning calories" is *not* the point of this exercise because calories have *nothing* to do with the hormonal problem, insulin resistance, that causes fat storage and high blood sugar. Focus on blunting blood sugar after meals through exercise, and your weight will come down because you are *controlling* your blood sugar and insulin levels through appropriate diet and functional exercise together.

Testing Your Blood Sugar

Buy a cheap blood sugar meter and test strips if you're prediabetic and test blood sugar regularly in the first 6 weeks to see what cause foods cause spikes, how exercise helps, and to help you adjust one or both. Ideal should be:

70-90 before eating (fasting)

No more than 120 at 2 hours after eating
(Ideally it should be back in the 70-90 range)

Test 8 times per day for the first 4 weeks in order to learn how your blood sugar responds to diet and exercise and to prevent spikes. For example, if you blood sugar is above 120 before you go to bed, do 10-20 minutes of brisk exercise, and you will lower it so that it's not high for several hours during the night exposing your organs and tissues to high sugar for 7-8 hours. Once you know what foods/drinks spike your blood sugar, then you know to avoid them.

Test at the following times:

When you first wake up
Before lunch
1 hour after lunch
2 hours after lunch
Before dinner
1 hour after dinner
2 hours after dinner
Before you go to bed.

Once you know which foods/drinks and in what amounts don't spike your blood sugar, then you can test at just 2 hours after meals to make sure your blood sugar is under 120, and the closer to 70-90 the better. Your blood sugar will be at its highest about 45 minutes to-1.5 hours after eating.

You can see how exercise drops your blood sugar by testing before and after exercising. Exercising after you eat blunts the rise in blood sugar. It's very useful to take your blood sugar at 1 hour after a meal, then exercise for 20 minutes, and take it again to see how much and which types of exercise drop it the most. It's trial and error, but you'll quickly get a sense of what works.

Ideal A1C is under 5.4, *and as close to 5.1 or 5.2 as possible*. Most MD's use the ADA guidelines and will tell you under 5.7 is normal. Metabolically, that's not the case. Data is showing that people with *5.4 and under* are metabolically normal; when A1C is over 5.4 the negative effects discussed above are happening and show up as high blood pressure, triglycerides, cholesterol, etc. even if A1C is under 5.7.

A1C is an *average* of 3 months of sugar bonded to the hemoglobin protein in the blood. It's an indirect measurement. *It does not show the variation in blood sugar from day to day or the number of damaging spikes or your level of insulin resistance*. So, A1C will not show all the spikes that harm blood vessels, prompt the liver to store glucose as fat, etc. Someone's A1C can be "normal" (under 5.7) because the insulin impairment is not as severe—*yet*—when blood sugar stays up constantly.

So they're getting very bad spikes with "normal" A1c under 5.7, but the blood sugar comes down eventually—just more and more slowly until it stops coming down. Ultimately, the blood sugar will stay high all the time—i.e. diabetes. It's only a matter of time for many people.

Daily testing and combining dietary changes and functional exercise to keep it within range, day after day, is *all about eliminating the spikes and decreasing the amount of insulin circulating in your body*. It's about stopping the damage these spikes and elevated insulin do over time. Do these things and your (A1C) will improve—and keep improving.

Food List, Shopping, and Basic Weekly Meal Prep

Spend the first week or two buying and stocking up on appropriate foods and starting a cooking routine. *Remember, the disease of insulin resistance drives hunger and food cravings and misalignment of insulin and cell receptors so glucose isn't getting into cells*—hence hunger. Remember that carbohydrate, especial sugar, is *very addictive*; protein and fat are not addictive, and these are the two *essential* macronutrients in the human diet. Carbohydrate is *optional.*

When you prepare and eat whole foods and don't eat processed foods, most grains, flours, or sugar you *remove excess calories, but you are not restricting calories*. This may seem like a subtle distinction, but you're removing the foods that cause the most serious problems metabolically; calories aren't the issue—biochemistry is the issue. A diet without processed food, grains, flours, and sugar means that you're removing the foods that do the most damage by raising blood sugar and insulin levels, which causes weight gain.

Once all the processed foods and drinks, grains and flours, sugars and fake sugars are gone, it's a lot more difficult to eat too much because our appetite evens out in response to removing these foods. On a low-carb diet we're far less hungry because we've gotten rid of the problem that's been driving excessive hunger. We can't get into too much trouble eating extra above ground veggies, protein, and fat, etc. My view is that if you're still hungry because your insulin resistance is still bad, have the extra portion of veggies, cheese, protein, etc. After a couple of months of eating this way and doing functional exercise every day you will no longer want the extra food. As your insulin sensitivity improves your hunger evens out—*a lot.*

It's astonishing how addictive the optional macronutrient carbohydrate is. Once we're no longer in the grip of a high carb/sugar diet, especially processed foods and all those supposedly "whole grains," it's *amazing* how even appetite becomes. We become hungry in a more gradual and natural way. Rarely, if ever, do we feel starving. If we exercise a lot, we can feel quite hungry, which is natural after hard exercise. That's very different from being hungry all the time, or needing to eat every couple of hours, or feeling "hangry," etc. These are all signs of carbohydrate withdrawal.

We can spend our entire lives feeling withdrawal symptoms from carbohydrate—i.e. feeling this multiple times a day. This is what a diet high in carbohydrate, especially refined and processed grains and flours, and too much sugar, does to us. It puts us in a constant state of chronic withdrawal. *This is due to evolution, not personal failings*. We don't get addicted to protein or to fat. We become addicted to carbohydrate very, very easily—some of us more than others. This is entirely because of how we evolved as humans over millions of years. We're *vulnerable* to carbohydrate as a species—all of us.

In essence, our relationship to carbohydrate determines blood sugar and insulin sensitivity. Genetics, exercise, sleep and stress all play supporting roles so to speak; the main character is, and always will be, carbohydrate. Thus, the treatment for a carbohydrate-driven disease, prediabetes and diabetes, is consuming whole, nutrient-dense foods, plenty of natural fat, and eliminating all the addictive, easily digestible carbs (flours, grains, and sugars) that drive up blood sugar, don't trigger release of our satiety hormones, and cause insulin resistance.

Dietary treatment of high blood sugar also means eliminating artificial sweeteners that trigger the body to go into insulin overdrive. For this to work, you *must* have the right foods available at all times. You must also be sure *not to have any of the foods/drinks available* that spike your blood sugar, such as refined carbohydrates (flours, sugars, grains), processed foods, juices, sugary fruits, etc.

Availability of the right foods and *not having any of the wrong foods available* as well as food preparation are the keys to everything.

Food Staples are those items you always have and from which you can make *many combinations* for meals. This list isn't very long because controlling high blood sugar and its underlying insulin resistance means eating real food that's complex and makes the body *work harder* to break it down. This means you have *ingredients* in the house, not processed or prepared foods that are ready to eat.

You might spend more on organic choices, but you will save a lot of money by not buying processed and prepared foods or juices or foods/drinks with artificial sweeteners such as diet sodas. Second, you will save *a lot of money long term* regarding the astronomical costs of high blood sugar and metabolic syndrome—especial money you won't need to spend on prescription drugs to "manage" these dietary diseases such as diabetes, hypertension, cholesterol problems etc.

You are now a connoisseur of food, a culinary adventurer! Getting rid of all processed and prepared foods means saving a lot of money *and* you have a great opportunity to try new things and new cuisines. Don't be intimidated! Great chefs experiment; it's what makes them great chefs.

You don't need a lot of ingredients to make many kinds of fantastic meals with real variety, and they don't need to take a lot of time to prepare. Spending a couple of hours a week prepping food is absolutely crucial. *Food prep* is the key to everything.

Basic Staples

Organic lentil or bean low-sodium soups in boxes or cans without BPA lining. You can extend these with rinsed canned beans and chopped veggies, broth, and herbs for soup that's fast and easy to make. Add the veggies you like, just use several kinds so you have a range of tastes, textures, and nutrients. Add some chicken or veggie broth, garlic, a good herb mixture, a little Parmesan cheese and olive oil, and you're all set. As always, use beans and legumes in very limited quantity until you know—via your blood testing on your meter—how they affect your blood sugar.

Organic fruit that's lower on the glycemic index such as berries, tomatoes, avocados, lemons and limes. Apples are high in carbohydrate, so eat half an apple at a time, and combine with peanut butter or cheese—i.e. fat to slow the absorption of the carbohydrate, especially the sugar. Don't forget about frozen berries. You can put frozen berries through a dessert maker for a wonderful sorbet that has no added sugar. The flavor is so intense you will only want to eat a small amount. Go slowly with fruit because of the natural sugar. If your blood sugar isn't coming down, eliminate all fruit until your blood sugar is better and your insulin sensitivity improved. You can use fresh lemon or lime for vitamin C.

Lemons can also be used in a variety of ways in cooking to bring brightness to a dish and provide valuable vitamin C without the sugar. I marinate fish in lemon and olive oil before cooking, which infuses it with that brightness. After baking the fish, I reduce the lemon and fish liquid from the cooked fish in a pan on high heat with butter and herbs, and strain it over the fish before serving.

This reduction technique can be used with almost any sauce, and it only takes a minute or two, but it creates a very complex flavor with some saturated fat in the butter to help with satiety and for helping our bodies absorb fat-soluble vitamins. If you heat up leftovers this reduction sauce keeps the fish moist and flavorful. You can cook 3-4 lbs. of fish (or meat or poultry) this way, depending on the size of your family, and this sauce will let you heat up leftovers without the fish becoming dry. This saves a lot of time.

Organic dairy such as creamer, butter, cheese, etc. Be very careful of yogurt. Even many "natural" yogurts have added sugar, fruit juice, etc., and there's a high level of natural sugar in milk/yogurt. Don't eat low fat yogurt—it has a high level of natural sugar without the fat to slow the absorption of that sugar. Until your blood sugar is stabilized and your insulin sensitivity improved, include some full fat dairy such as cheese and heavy cream in your coffee; these won't spike blood sugar very much.

Organic meat (e.g. chicken, red meat, turkey, organ meats)

Organic canned tomatoes for making many kinds of dishes.

Organic broth, low sodium, for soups and to use as flavoring in dishes. (If you can, freeze the bones from your meats and make your own broth. If you have a slow cooker, this is easy to do, and you get all the minerals from the bones.)

Organic mushrooms, which are *powerful* immune boosters—even the plain white button mushrooms!

Organic beans/legumes—dried or canned without BPA lining to make soups, chili, use in sauces for extra fiber, to make cold bean salads with chopped veggies, etc.

Organic eggs

Organic greens—use the boxed or bagged kind. Supermarkets use chemicals in the sprayers over the produce section. Boxes/bags protects the greens.

Hummus, organic if possible

Organic veggies whenever possible, and buy seasonally for better deals. Never eat conventional celery or red peppers or broccoli or kale—they are some of the worst and most toxic crops—eat only organic with these. Focus on a range of colors and those veggies that grow above ground because they have far less starch. You should have enough veggies to eat at lunch and dinner.

Don't forget about **frozen veggies**, which have good nutritional profiles. Peas, onions, organic broccoli, etc. are all great frozen choices because you can just add them to soups without chopping. Having a variety in the freezer always means you have things to add to soups or to other dishes. Use peas and onions in moderation as they have more starch.

Always have garlic and herbs on hand to add to soups and a variety of dishes. If garlic is too pungent, you can roast whole cloves along with your veggies/meat/ fish, and that way you can spread it on the final dish. Roasted garlic has a much sweeter taste. Using crushed garlic in soups adds to the robustness, and if you don't use a lot, it won't take over the flavor profile.

You can roast a whole, red onion as a vegetable, and it tastes very sweet and makes a wonderful side for meat or beans—again in very limited portions because it's not an above ground vegetable, but it has a lot less sugar than potatoes or carrots, etc.

Quinoa, Nuts, Chia Seeds, and Ground flax for fiber and omega 3 fatty acids. Quinoa is a complete protein; it is high in carbohydrate, so be sure you're testing your blood sugar to see if you can tolerate it. Be sure to get ground flax seeds as humans can't digest whole flax seeds, so we don't get the benefits of the omega 3 fatty acids. Keep ground flax in the fridge in a dark bag or container.

Wild salmon whenever possible or other kinds of fatty fish. Used canned wild salmon when fresh is out of season. When wild salmon is available in season and on sale, get extra to freeze. You can mix previously-frozen wild salmon with an egg and herbs of your choice to make wild salmon cakes that are great hot or cold. I advise against farm-raised salmon, which does not have the same nutritional profile as wild salmon in terms of omega-3 fatty acids. Better to get wild on sale and freeze it to make salmon cakes later.

Sardines make a fast, affordable snack or light meal that won't spike your blood sugar. They provide lots of bioavailable calcium if you eat the bones. They're very economical and stay shelf stable for years. The wild sardines are best. They're also low on the food chain, so they're not building up mercury and other toxins in their flesh the way larger fish can such as tuna.

Herbs, dried or fresh. Some herbs such as oregano have far more antioxidants when dry. Think in terms of creating several herb mixes that you can put together in separate containers for quick use in creating a complex flavor profile to any dish, e.g. basil, oregano, thyme, rosemary and bay for dishes such as meatballs with chopped tomatoes, olive oil, and red onion.

A range of spice mixes and marinades, etc. that you like, which are low in sugar and salt. The Teeny Tiny Spice Company has an excellent line of organic spice mixes that you can just add quickly to meat, fish, or veggies to make a dish with a complex flavor profile without all the work. They have choices of spice mixes from all over the world; meals do not have to be dreary, bland affairs to reduce your blood sugar.

Often I add a tablespoon or two of my favorite of these spice mixes to Greek yogurt to marinate chicken, fish, and meat, which adds calcium and fat—don't use low fat yogurt! Be sure to get yogurt that does not have any added sugar or sweeteners. The marinade should cling to the chicken or fish or meat so it's coated when it goes in the oven at 325 degrees. This marinade ensures the chicken, or fish, or meat stays moist so you can cook a substantial amount ahead of time and just reheat quickly for subsequent meals.

Organic olive oil and vinegars

Use the money you were spending on processed/prepared foods to get a single-source, extra-virgin organic olive oil. It will be more expensive, but it's a good fat that is stable at the molecular level when heated. "Vegetable" oils such as canola, corn, safflower, etc. come from intensive industrial processes and are not stable, nor can our bodies process them properly.

Try different vinegars. As a fermented food, vinegar has real health benefits, particularly for gut health. There's good quality options that are worth the money, and you will be saving money when you don't purchase processed/prepared foods, which are very expensive.

Cooking and Weekly Food Prep

Cook a large tray of cut veggies once or twice per week depending on the size of your family. This way you'll always have plenty of variety, sufficient micronutrients, and sufficient carbs for energy that don't spike blood sugar in the way refined carbs do. Chop, toss with olive oil or butter and herbs, and cook in oven on 325 degrees (not too hot), lower rack, with some water so they don't dry out. Cook until just tender.

Cook dense veggies like cauliflower and Brussels sprouts together on one tray and more fragile veggies like peppers, mushrooms, etc. on another tray, as they'll be different cooking times. You can mix with dressing (olive oil and vinegar—not soybean oil!!) for a cold dish. You can eat these veggies as is, or add to soup, or toss with a spice mix you like, or use as part of another dish such as the chicken, fish, meat in the spiced yogurt marinade I described above. This means you get several dinners of meat, fish, chicken and a wide variety of veggies for several days—saving a lot of time in getting dinner on the table.

Spend 1 hour cutting and prepping the veggies for these tray bakes depending on the size of your family. When they're cooked and ready in the fridge, you'll find yourself eating lot more veggies! Don't overcook your trays of veggies. That way you can heat them up easily for meals during the week without drying them out or making them too soft.

Get portions of organic/natural meats/fish for the week, and go with what's on sale whenever possible, using your freezer to store deals you find. Use canned sardines and wild salmon to supplement in weeks when fish isn't on sale. When good meat is on sale, buy extra to freeze.

You can marinate skinless chicken or meat or fish in full-fat, unsweetened yogurt into which you have stirred in herbs/seasoning of your choice. Bake at 325 degrees. The yogurt seals in all the juices and flavoring of the seasonings you've added. (This is the method of making tandoori meat and fish in north Indian food.) You can bake chicken and meat and fish with a variety of marinades (without sugar), herbs, butter, etc. You can cook fish with lemon and herbs or a variety of marinades or dry herb mixes.

Make a soup weekly with organic beans/lentils, veggies, and meat (if you eat meat). I make a soup on Friday or Saturday using remaining veggies in the fridge and from the tray bakes, which means I never throw anything out, and we have fast meals during busy weekends. All the veggies and meat gets used at the end of the week. Food is expensive, so it's important that everything gets eaten, and food waste is a *big contributor* to global warming.

End-of-week soup is a great way to use everything and use your homemade broth. Toss in fresh herbs and greens such as spinach or kale at the very end of cooking for added nutrients and flavor. You can add quinoa for texture and protein if your blood sugar can tolerate the carbohydrate, just make the quinoa ahead of time and stir it in at the very end or after you've turned off the heat.

If you want to make traditional hummus and your blood sugar can tolerate it, it's very easy and takes 5 minutes, and it's *much* cheaper than buying it. (Regular hummus: two cans of well-rinsed, organic, garbanzo beans (chickpeas), lemon juice, tahini, garlic bulb or two, and olive oil to taste, put in blender and blast away until smooth. Done!) I make white bean hummus, black bean hummus, regular hummus, hummus with cooked veggies such as red pepper from weekly tray bake, red lentil hummus, etc.) You can make hummus out of anything. Avocado hummus is delicious too!

Make extra portions of your hummus, tomato sauces, etc. to freeze. Because you aren't eating processed or prepared foods, it's important to use your time efficiently by prepping for the entire week so you can just pull dinner together quickly. Freeze 2-3 portions of your soup so that you always have something you can pull out of the freezer for dinner if needed.

Eating

Use smaller bowls/plates—which encourages you to pace yourself. It takes about 20 minutes for the food we eat to signal to our brains that we're getting full—this has to do with how long it takes for food to get to a certain place in our digestive system, which then signals the brain. Smaller plates remind us to eat what we have slowly so we wait for the hormonal signals of satiety to kick in before automatically eating more.

This 20-minute delay between when we start putting food in our mouths and when the brain starts to register fullness can cause us to eat too much too quickly—and then feel "stuffed."

If your blood sugar can tolerate them, eat beans/legumes most days along with some protein, fat, veggies (mostly above ground veggies and leafy greens), limited fruit (berries, avocado, tomato), and nuts/seeds. I would advise eating veggies and fat at every meal to help with nutrients and fiber and feeling full throughout your day.

Have good snacks available (protein or protein/fat combination) if needed in first few weeks. After that, you'll notice the need for snacks decreases as your insulin resistance improves. Better to snack on real food, which triggers the hormones that tell us we're full. After a while, you'll find that as your blood sugar stabilizes and your insulin improves, you will need to snack less often. This will happen naturally, and it's a sign that your blood sugar and insulin levels are improving. The hunger will start to subside as your insulin sensitivity improves because your cells are getting the glucose they need.

If you have to have a snack—*eat a protein/fat/fiber combination.* Don't eat carbs alone or that will spike your blood sugar. Blood sugar stays relatively constant during the night except in the very early morning, usually between 2:00-7:00 a.m. when the liver dumps stored sugar to help us wake up. There's also a release of hormones that increases insulin resistance, which causes blood sugar to rise.

High morning blood sugar may also be caused by a carbohydrate snack at night. So, don't drive your blood sugar up at night before going to bed with a carb snack because that's a 7-8 hour period of high blood sugar! Eat nuts, protein, or cheese if you need a snack that won't spike your blood sugar.

Conclusion

A diagnosis of prediabetes can be devastating and confusing, particularly if you're already eating what we've been told for decades is a healthy diet—low in fat (especially saturated fat), high in "whole grains" and other carbs lumped together under "fruits and vegetables" as if these were all the same, lean meat and poultry, "vegetable" oils, etc.

From a metabolic health as well as an evolutionary perspective, this is not a healthy diet. It's far better than the standard American diet of 60% processed foods, desserts, sugary drinks, artificial sweeteners, etc.—the most toxic diet on the face of the earth.

This seemingly healthy diet of "whole grains," lots of fruits, lean protein, starchy carbs, too little natural fat, and toxic "vegetable" oils is not what our bodies are designed to eat on a constant basis, and the pandemic of chronic metabolic health problems shows us this. It can be very dispiriting to feel we've been eating the right things, but we develop prediabetes anyway. The problem lies in the fact that we've been *told the wrong things* for decades.

It's especially disheartening if we have tried to lower blood sugar by controlling our weight using a calorie-reduction diet because we've been told the "formula" of calories in/calories out is akin to a law of nature. It is not. It's a narrative, a metaphor for energy that does not apply to the human body and never did.

Reducing calories can trick the body for 6 months or so into losing weight; however, given how much the human body prioritizes fat for survival, the body resets itself in response to what it perceives as starvation, and our metabolism slows down. Then we gain the weight back and more. The way we lose weight is the same way we control blood sugar; eat below our carbohydrate tolerance and restore our insulin sensitivity.

As a society we've made carbohydrate, an optional macronutrient, the center of our agricultural economy, and giant processed food companies have controlled the discourses about food and health for far too long—including through all the research they fund and the groups they support that advocate a diet high in carbohydrate, including plenty of "whole grains"—when absolutely anything can and is called a "whole grain."

Yet, we have removed one of the two essential macronutrients, fat, from just about everything—including from the animals themselves through changes in breeding. We have created monstrous "plant-based" oils out of the toxic and dangerous byproducts of other industries in order to make more profits—telling people they must consume these light machine oils because the natural sources of fat that we have eaten for millions of years suddenly became dangerous to the human species in the late twentieth century. Nonsense!

A diagnosis of prediabetes is an enormously valuable opportunity to prevent progression to Type 2 diabetes and its complications. By reversing the root cause of most cases of prediabetes, which is insulin resistance—sometimes in conjunction with hyperinsulinemia—you're also reversing the cause of the entire cluster of metabolic diseases and conditions known a "metabolic syndrome," including high blood pressure, weight, and cholesterol problems.

By addressing the imbalance in the hormone insulin at the root of the problem, you can reverse blood sugar, weight, blood pressure, and cholesterol problems. Doing so means you're changing the course of your health in profound ways—lowering significantly your risk of cardiovascular disease, nonalcoholic fatty liver disease, dementia, and some cancers.

Begin where you are.

You don't need fancy recipes to make great meals. Get the ingredients/staples in this guide and experiment. *Learn to trust your sense of food; we all have it.* You don't need to be a trained chef, but you do need to be willing to prepare food in an organized way and plan ahead. Your freezer is your friend! Make double and store it! If you use high quality ingredients, you don't need a lot of food because excellent (organic if possible), whole, and complex ingredients taste *much better* and they *signal to our bodies tha we're full*. They also taste far better than processed foods, which use the cheapest ingredients possible (including cheap "vegetable" oils) in order to maximize their profits, cheap ingredients that destroy our health and trigger our evolutionary vulnerabilities such as carb and sugar cravings.

Processed foods don't tell us we're full because they evade our natural hormonal signals that tell us we're full. (Processed foods are *designed* to do this so that we keep eating them.) Real, complex, whole foods align with our hormonal systems because that's what we ate as a species for millions of years. Eating the 3 macronutrients together—protein, fat, and good carbs—at every meal signals to our bodies that we're full. When we get these satiety signals it becomes a lot harder to eat too much, and we don't want to do so!

Get creative with herbs, spice mixes, marinades without sugar or "vegetable" oils, and combinations of foods such as tossing a few blueberries into a savory dish. Cooking enough soup and other dishes to freeze means if you get sick or are extremely busy you have enough in the freezer for several meals.

In terms of exercise, you don't need a gym membership or expensive workout clothing. Walk around the parking lot before and after errands, walk up and down stairs, carry groceries out to your car, and take short but brisk walks after meals. Do some squats and modified pushups against the wall and use a set of dumbbells that are appropriate a few times a week (i.e. resistance training.) When you walk, speed up for one minute, then walk at normal pace for 1 minute, and repeat. This, too, is HIIT. Done consistently these exercises will make a huge difference in blunting your blood sugar after meals, throughout the day, and at night when you're sleeping.

Test your blood sugar so you know which foods trigger blood sugar spikes and how you can best keep your blood sugar at 120 or below 2 hours after a meal, preferably lower. <u>At 140 or above, blood sugar does damage in the body</u>, so target that 120 maximum (lower whenever possible) two hours after eating and 70-90 before meals.

Don't go to bed with high blood sugar. Do one or two 10-minute bursts of exercise until your blood sugar comes down to the 70-90 range so that you spend 7-8 hours of your day asleep with good blood sugar. That's 30% of your day, and it makes a *huge difference* in terms of increasing your insulin sensitivity and preventing your body from storing high blood sugar as fat.

Work *with your body's natural hormonal signals*. These signals *will* tell you you're full—provided that you're eating real, whole foods and not processed/high carb foods such as white potatoes, wheat, corn, or natural sugar such as honey or fruit with high sugar content, or artificial sweeteners.

Create ways to get functional exercise throughout your day, and work up to 30 minutes of exercise in one session. Do activities that strengthen your muscles and make your heart work. It won't take long before you can do more resistance training and HIIT, and there are a lot of great resources to help you when you're ready.

Finally, remember that getting enough sleep and reducing stress as much as possible will significantly help in lowering your blood sugar and insulin levels.

Remember, you can reverse prediabetes. Doing so will change the course of your life!

Other Books in the Metabolic Health Publications Series

Written by an historian of science, this series provides the general reader with a range of accessible books and guides regarding metabolic health.

Our Metabolic Health Crisis: An In-Depth Guide to Reversing Insulin Resistance, Prediabetes/Type 2 Diabetes, Weight, Blood Pressure, and Cholesterol Problems

Insulin resistance is the massive, silent epidemic driving the vast majority of chronic health problems. Written by an historian of science, *Our Metabolic Health Crisis* is a comprehensive resource for the general reader who wants to reverse insulin resistance and the chronic diseases and conditions it causes, diseases and conditions that now affect 88% of American adults:

- prediabetes and Type 2 diabetes
- weight gain and obesity
- nonalcoholic fatty liver disease (NAFLD)
- high blood pressure
- cholesterol problems including high triglycerides

Our Metabolic Health Crisis leads you through the 7 science-based steps that reverse insulin resistance, Metabolic Syndrome, as well as many other conditions that have insulin resistance at their root. Taking the 7 steps in *Our Metabolic Health Crisis* that reverse insulin resistance also means you also decrease systemic inflammation, support your immune system, improve vascular and liver health, and lower your risk of the many weight-associated cancers driven by high glucose and insulin levels in the body.

Reversing insulin resistance is what *promotes* weight loss and the ability to keep the weight off over time. Weight loss is about increasing insulin sensitivity, not counting calories, or worrying about dietary fat, or trying to "burn" enough calories, etc. A key reason for this is that high insulin levels *prevent cells from releasing fatty acids—i.e. too much insulin works like a hormonal lock preventing cells from releasing fat*. Weight loss is essentially a hormonal process, i.e. it's not about counting or burning calories, etc.

Only diet and food timing (when you eat) affect the cellular pathways of insulin resistance. Unlike medications to "manage" but not reverse dietary diseases, or drugs that make them worse such as exogenous insulin for Type 2 diabetes, the effective diet and food-timing steps in *Our Metabolic Health Crisis* don't cost anything. The 7 achievable steps in *Our Metabolic Health Crisis* also improve cardiovascular, brain, liver, and immune health because each is profoundly affected by insulin resistance.

Our Metabolic Health Crisis also includes valuable tools and resources for understanding insulin resistance and the chronic diseases and conditions it causes and drives. J. Smythe-Rivers explains the most important tests to discuss with your doctors, including insulin resistance tests and the coronary calcium scan, which is the best predictor of heart attack risk for most people.

Finally, *Our Metabolic Health Crisis* gives the reader curated, free, online, expert resources in metabolic, cardiovascular, and brain health to use and share with family and friends. *Our Metabolic Health Crisis* makes a wonderful gift too.

The Only Diet You'll Ever Need: Insulin Resistance, Leptin Resistance, and Weight Loss

If you've tried diets in the past or you're considering a diet now, *The Only Diet You'll Ever Need* is for you. Many diets provide weight loss at first, but over time we almost always gain the weight back. This happens because most diets don't reverse the actual reasons we put on weight and have difficulty keeping it off, which are insulin resistance and leptin resistance. We can have one or both hormonal imbalances.

Losing weight and keeping it off permanently is about correcting these two diet-driven hormonal problems, not worrying about calories, fat, meat, or dairy. You can control your insulin and leptin levels whether you eat meat, or you're a vegetarian, flexitarian, or vegan.

Written by historian of science J. Smythe-Rivers, *The Only Diet You'll Ever Need* gives you the key, science-based dietary steps to take that reverse insulin resistance and leptin resistance so you lose the weight—and gain many other health benefits such as better blood sugar, better blood pressure, and better cholesterol levels.

The Only Diet You'll Ever Need is not a recipe book. It is the ideal overview for anyone who wants to understand why we gain weight, why appetite increases in response to these hormonal problems, and how to lose weight safely and effectively by reversing the two causes of weight gain, which are hormonal not caloric.

Before you start any diet, or if you're currently on a diet now, read *The Only Diet You'll Ever Need*, which guides you through these two diet-driven hormonal problems causing weight gain as well as how to lose weight safely and permanently. *The Only Diet You'll Ever Need* also makes a wonderful gift.

A Very Brief History of the Low-Carb and Keto Diet

In this very short history of the low-carb and ketogenic diets, historian of science J. Smythe-Rivers provides an informative interpretation of William Banting's nineteenth-century pamphlet, "Letter on Corpulence, Addressed to the Public," which is the first text on the low-carb diet. She provides the historical and medical roots of the ketogenic diet as well as a succinct explanation of how the keto diet works. This brief guide to the history of the low-carb and keto movements is an ideal gift for the beginner exploring these diets or for anyone interested in these topics.

12 Habits that Control Blood Sugar and Reverse Prediabetes is a habit-based guide for those with elevated blood sugar or prediabetes as well as for those who would like to keep their normal blood sugar from rising. This guide is also useful for those with Type 2 diabetes who would like a quick set of reminders about diet and exercise that are proven to lower blood sugar.

Chapters cover an overview of prediabetes and diabetes, A1C, and insulin resistance; testing blood sugar; eating the right carbohydrates; removing sugar(s) from your diet; the importance of making fiber-filled and micronutrient-rich food substitutions; artificial sweeteners and insulin resistance; fiber as critical to gut micro biome health, insulin sensitivity, and lowering blood sugar; the importance of preparing your own meals as part of controlling blood sugar and saving money; daily functional exercise with an overview of strength training and HIIT; the relationship between sleep and blood sugar; and reducing stress.

The 6 Habits for Losing Weight provides an overview and discussion of 6 critical habits for losing weight and improving metabolic health, including lowering blood sugar, blood pressure, and cholesterol. Consumption of refined grains has risen steadily over the past 50 years, and this guide provides an historical framework for weight loss as a matter of removing that dietary excess rather than counting calories.

Other chapters cover the importance of balancing macro- and micronutrients for weight loss, removing the excess sedentary behavior that has increased significantly in recent decades, the importance of fiber in weight loss, the dangers of sleep deprivation vis-à-vis weight gain, and the significance of developing one's insulin sensitivity as part of losing weight and improving metabolic health.

In ***Prediabetes: A Patient's Guide to Preventing Diabetes,*** Smyth-Rivers provides a distilled overview of prediabetes and diabetes, insulin resistance, high blood pressure and cholesterol, and weight loss. She gives you the diet and exercise plans that will lower blood sugar to normal, increase insulin sensitivity, and stabilize blood pressure and cholesterol. These dietary and exercise plans will result in weight loss, which is the direct result of controlled blood sugar and increased insulin sensitivity.

Losing weight is not a matter of simple willpower; it's a matter of hormones. The staple foods and methods of eating Smythe-River provides in this book signal the satiety hormone (leptin), so it becomes difficult to overeat. Drawing on current science and dietary research in diabetes prevention, Smythe-Rivers provides the 10 essential dietary steps that reverse high blood sugar and signal satiety. She provides valuable insight into the ways in which food order, food combinations, and food timing affect blood sugar. Smythe-Rivers covers the critical importance of dietary micronutrients (not supplements) in blunting hunger, balancing blood sugar, and reducing inflammation.

Smythe-Rivers provides readers with a concise grocery list of widely available staples from which to make delicious meals quickly, meals that will build insulin sensitivity and reverse prediabetes. She shows you why these staple foods and methods of eating align with our bodies from an evolutionary perspective, which means they also signal satiety, and we no longer want to eat too much. Her list of staple foods and methods of eating also give you the crucial flexibility and choices you need, not an inflexible diet or one that relies on complicated ingredients.

Smythe-Rivers provides readers with a detailed discussion of functional exercise, strength training, and HIIT (High-Intensity Interval Training) as well as important information about the A1C test and when to test your blood sugar as part of reversing prediabetes. In addition to diet and exercise, she addresses two equally important factors that drive high blood sugar: stress and lack of sleep.

My Daily Journal: Blood Sugar, Food, and Exercise

This journal is a companion to the books in the Metabolic Health Publications series to help you track your blood sugar, sleep, food, and exercise on a daily basis for 16 weeks. At the end of each week you also track your achievements for the week and your goals for the forthcoming week. You create your shopping list of food items for the following week based on the list of staples in the book *Prediabetes: A Patient's Guide to Preventing Diabetes*. There is also room each week for you to make additional notes about your progress and questions.

This journal is specifically designed to follow the plan for stabilizing and reversing prediabetes in *Prediabetes: A Patient's Guide to Preventing Diabetes*; however, you can also use this journal with other the books in the Metabolic Health Publications series or as part of your own plan to address prediabetes or Type 2 diabetes.

Stop Counting Calories to Lose Weight!

In this brief but fascinating guide, historian of science Josie Smythe-Rivers shows you why counting calories is the enemy of weight loss.

Calories don't matter to the body. The body has no receptors for "calories." Calories tell us nothing about what our bodies do with what we eat and drink. While we are busy counting calories and worrying unnecessarily about the fats in food, our bodies metabolize what we eat and drink through biochemical and hormonal processes and pathways. The body does not recognize, use, or burn calories. Counting calories keeps us constantly hungry, and counting calories can harm our health both metabolically and nutritionally.

Initially weight loss can happen on many kinds of diets--up to a point--and then we regain the weight we lost and more. The reason for this is when we lose weight strong evolutionary and hormonal factors slow our metabolism, increase our hunger, and decrease our satiety in response to that weight loss. Further, we become more (not less) tempted by foods and our ability to resist them declines. Because of these evolutionary responses to weight loss, keeping the weight off over time is impossible using the calories-in/calories-out model (CICO), which decades of studies have demonstrated. Thus, we end up trying to restrict calories even more, but despite doing so we put the weight back on.

In addition to her brief, fascinating history of the calorie and its misapplication to the human body and nutrition science, Smythe-Rivers provides readers with the 6 steps that ensure long-term weight loss based on how our bodies actually work in terms evolutionary biology, including our hormones. She also addresses why metabolism slows and hunger increases in response to weight loss; most importantly, she addresses how to overcome these facts to avoid gaining the weight back.

Excerpts:

"The human body is not a steam engine, and it doesn't consume or use energy like one. The human body does not function in the ways that objects or phenomena do that physicists study. Yet, the very notion of a "calorie" in nutrition science was inaccurately transposed from these other realms of science as a metaphorical way of trying to talk about how we consume and use energy."

"When we pretend "calories in/calories out" is a real equation we encourage people to ignore why they're gaining weight in the first place, why we have difficulty losing weight, and more importantly, why decades of studies show it's so difficult to keep it off over time. The dubious 'equation' and model of calories in/calories out (CICO) blames the person who fails to keep weight off because she or he failed to 'eat less and move more.' Exercise is wonderful for us, but it has very little to do with weight loss. Counting calories ignores the fact that we metabolize different foods very differently, and they affect our health and weight very differently. We may talk and think in terms calories, but our bodies "speak" an entirely different language, the language of carbohydrates, lipids, and proteins."

"So, how do we lose weight and keep it off? We change what we're eating and when we're eating so that we're satiated by the foods we eat according to how our individual bodies metabolize those foods. We work with our biochemistry, not against it. The last two sections of this guide go into detail about what you should and shouldn't eat in relation to how the body actually works in terms of weight loss."

The Rivers Code: The 2 Steps to Losing Weight and Keeping it Off!

Diets based on the idea of "eat less/move more" and the misleading "formula" of "calories-in/calories-out" have been around since the Victorian period. They didn't work then, and they don't work now. Despite all the advances in modern medicine, when it comes to weight loss we're still being told to follow the same 19th-century, Victorian-age dieting advice.

The science has been clear for decades that the "calories-in/calories-out" dogma does not work because people regain the weight they've lost—and more. One can't restrict calories forever, and excellent studies since the mid-20th century have proven this.

Our bodies are designed to *resist weight loss* when we count calories. When we restrict calories our hunger increases; our metabolism slows down; our capacity to resist food decreases; and we become more sedentary. These are the body's ways of stopping weight loss based on calorie counting, which the body understands as famine and starvation.

Written by an historian of science, this short guide cuts through the nonsense about calorie counting as well as elaborate diets that are just different forms of calorie counting. Smythe-Rivers also outlines the ways in which corruption, greed, and remarkably bad science intentionally drive obesity and metabolic disease globally, especially through the 5 "big offender" foods that have infiltrated our lives and diets, often without our knowing it.

You don't need a complex and expensive diet program (e.g. prepared meals, supplements, etc.) to lose weight safely and effectively—if you make just 2 changes. Smythe-Rivers' 2-step program is not a diet; it removes the two primary problems that cause weight gain and prevent permanent weight loss.

The 2 steps are:

1.) Eliminate the 5 “big offender” foods that cause the weight gain in the first place, do the most damage to our metabolic health (e.g. diabetes, insulin resistance, leptin resistance, high cholesterol, high blood pressure, etc.), cholesterol, blood pressure), and cause us to regain the weight we lose.

2.) Time your eating to align with your biochemistry and human circadian rhythms.

In Step One Smythe-Rivers shows you why these 5 “big offender” foods that permeate every area of our lives are the direct cause of nearly all weight gain and poor metabolic health including diabetes, obesity, insulin resistance, heart disease, chronic inflammation, and brain/ cognitive disorders.

In Step Two, Smythe-Rivers gives you the specific window of time for eating nutrient-dense, healthy, and delicious meals that leave you full and satisfied—and most importantly that don’t restrict calories, slow your metabolism, or make you hungry the way counting calories always does.

You don’t need elaborate, expensive, restrictive, complicated, or frustrating diets. The 2-step process Smythe-Rivers has created aligns with your biochemistry and your circadian rhythms to prompt safe, effective weight loss that will significantly improve your metabolic health, including your blood sugar and insulin sensitivity, and allow you to keep the weight off permanently.

Printed in Great Britain
by Amazon

59922878R00102